HAPPINESS
WITHIN
THE SKIN

With the assistance
of Galya Ortega

JEAN-LOUIS POIROUX

HAPPINESS WITHIN THE SKIN

THE SECRETS OF HOLISTIC BEAUTY

ABRAMS | NEW YORK

CONTENTS

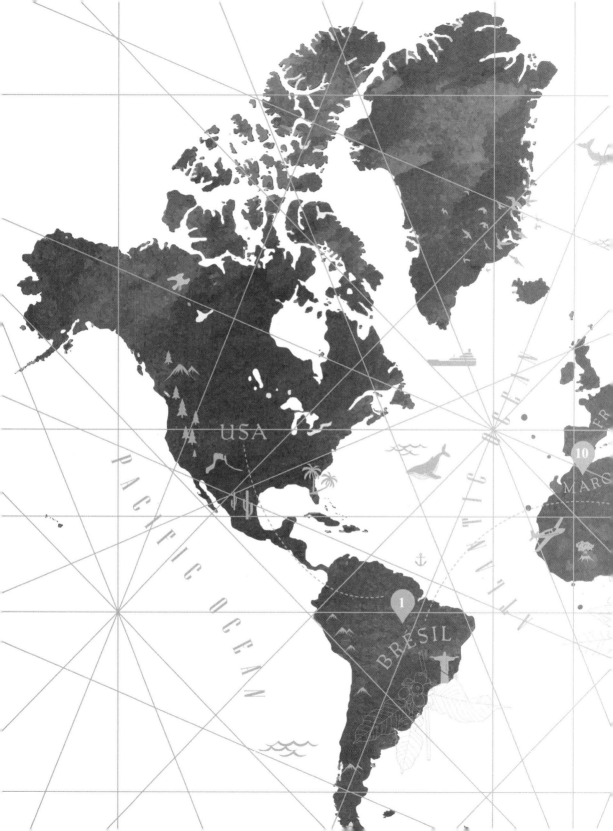

INTRODUCTION

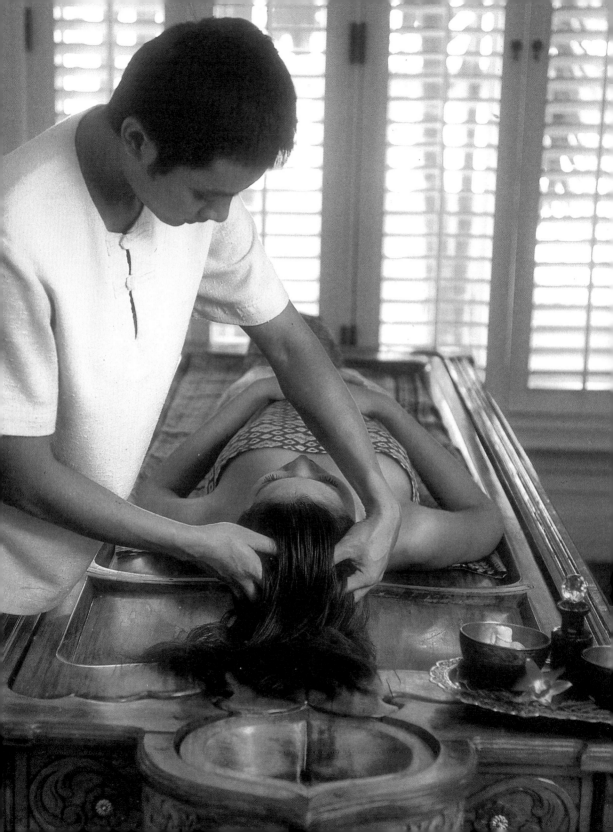

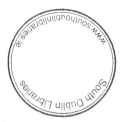

> *"The chief good is health,*
> *beauty is the second, wealth is the third"*
>
> PLATO

S ome vocations are so deeply rooted in our psyche that we are unaware of them at a conscious level. It is only when they emerge, shaped by time to become a compelling call to action, that we realize they existed all along.

So it was with my vocation, whose seeds were sown in 1988 when I first discovered Indian Ayurvedic massage while on military service in London, England. But it was another 13 years before I opened my first spa and launched the Cinq Mondes cosmetic range – 13 years that almost invisibly gave me the keys to unlock my future. You could say that in that time I assembled the pieces of the puzzle at the root of what is today, in 2018, an enterprise committed to wellness and beauty, with outlets in 36 countries and more than 1,000 Cinq Mondes spa partners worldwide.

This book aims to reveal the secrets of wellness and beauty – share the knowledge gained from working alongside practitioners of traditional medicine such as Ayurvedic and Chinese doctors and Balinese healers. All of their practice is based on a holistic approach, covering diet, the subtle interplay between body and mind but also skin nutrition. Because it is only when these three dimensions are in harmony that the expression "feeling comfortable in your own skin" makes any sense. Only then does a person's overall beauty really shine through.

Bringing those three dimensions together is key to the Cinq Mondes ethos. By taking this holistic approach to beauty, each one of our spas offers a place to re-energize and cultivate the art of wellness.

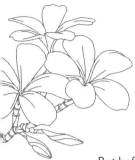

THE DAWNING
OF A PASSION

But before I go any further, let me begin by explaining what first kindled this passion of mine for self-awareness, inner balance, wellness and in the end, beauty.

Strangely enough, my fascination with such things started very early on. Hence my attraction, as a 19-year old fresh out of school and newly arrived in London, to "Asia Minor" – the nickname for Bayswater on account of the number of Indians who congregate there. I soon found myself knocking on the door of an Ayurvedic Centre and getting my very first warm sesame oil massage. This was in 1988 when hardly anyone in France had heard of Ayurveda, least of all my 900 fellow students at HEC Paris. My London friends, meanwhile, expressed serious reservations about so-called "Ayurvedic massage" ...

In fact, the *Abhyanga* (oil massage) is an integral part of a healing system that has been practiced on the Indian subcontinent for 5,000 years. Abhyanga massage works on both mind and body – hardly surprising therefore that it is now so popular with western consumers.

Equally strange in those days were my weekly visits to an aromatherapy center in Primrose Hill where I learned the healing powers of essential oils and the subtle balancing effects of Bach flower remedies. Not what you would expect of a young man of 19 certainly, but a sure sign of the passionate advocate for holistic wellness and beauty that I would become.

To complete the picture, I spent my military service with L'Oreal, where I would remain for 10 years learning about cosmetics manufacturing.

FATE
INTERVENES

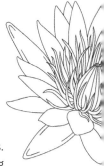

To be honest though, I didn't just study Ayurveda, aromatherapy and cosmetics. I also spent a lot of time "down the pub" knocking back pints in beer-drinking contests, partying with the rest of the French expat community in London and, of course, getting to know English girls of my age ...

So why this strange interest in massage and aromatherapy when nothing about my family or background tended that way? I think everyone has their own little idiosyncrasies – mine happened to be an innate awareness of tactile and olfactory sensations. What fascinated me at L'Oreal was the texture of the cosmetics, how they felt on the skin, and also fragrance development – that for me was as much a source of curiosity as a sheer olfactory delight.

But my career might never have taken off if not for ... jaundice. Hepatitis B to be precise. Not me, but another French conscript working at L'Oreal who had to be suddenly whisked home to France – a devastating turn of events for him but an absolute godsend for me. Suddenly the hunt was on to find his replacement.

I never met my unwitting benefactor because my first job on graduating from HEC was with a leading financial services company in Paris – so about as far as you can get from the perfume and cosmetics business. For three months I learned how to record numbers in debit and credit columns, double-checking the figures as I went, and carry out stocktaking. One particular client was a bolts manufacturer in Garonor on the outskirts of Paris. My job, perched at the top of interminable ladders, was to count every bolt destined for the aeronautical industry. Each one had a unit price of 37,000 francs – I remember the figure exactly – so I was told to be extra careful about counting them!

I went from there to stocktaking in an industrial sponge warehouse, still working for the same company in Paris where the associate director's one claim to fame was to have ordered the opening of sealed containers so she could blow the whistle on the shady accounting practices of a big company …

By the end of those three months, I was a broken man. One morning (for the first and only time in my entire life) I arrived at work with tears in my eyes. That was the day the call came through from L'Oreal's HRM and saved my bacon.

You could say that fate intervened – jaundice was the turning point that allowed me to create Cinq Mondes and I can't resist here drawing a parallel with this quote from the German poet Hölderlin: "The greater the danger, the greater the power of redemption."

FIVE DECISIVE
CROSSROADS

Looking back today, there were clearly five other major turning points in my life – five key moments, decisions or encounters that triggered my move toward entrepreneurship, starting at age 35 with the opening of the first French spa centered on traditions of wellness and beauty from around the world, and the launch of a cosmetics range that would underpin the entire business.

The first key moment came at the end of my first year of prepa at the Lycée Clemenceau in Nantes. Though I was admitted to the Ecole de Commerce Supérieure in Lyon, I turned it down in favor of repeating the year and trying for HEC. It was not the obvious choice given that no pupil from the school had ever made it into HEC before, but something inside told me it was a risk worth taking. A year later, I was admitted to HEC – an elite professional school where I lived on campus for three fascinating years and built a network of contacts that still serve me well today.

That – HEC – brought me my second big break. Because without that degree I would never have got a job with L'Oreal in London and with it, the opportunity to cultivate my passion for the beauty and wellness business. It was there that I met the executive vice-president of L'Oreal, Patrick Rabain, who headhunted me a few years later to take charge of developing a new range of hair-care products for Laboratoires Garnier. Three years of R&D led to the launch of Fructis, which was soon selling all over the world.

Following that success I was appointed director of new product development for L'Oreal hair-care products, a position that involved traveling to other European cities but also to the USA, Japan, Brazil and other places. That's how I came to discover American and Oriental spas and formed the idea for a French take on the spa culture – a temple of contemporary wellness and beauty French-style.

To flesh out that idea, I needed to become an entrepreneur myself – a wholly personal endeavor not without its risks within a big company. For that, I needed an intermediary stage.

It was just then that I met Philippe Champion, co-founder of the TAG Heuer luxury watch brand, who asked me to take over from him as international marketing director of the company. It meant leaving the world of beauty and wellness but it was a chance to learn from the best: high-achieving entrepreneurs in luxury goods who knew their business inside out. Store design, press and public relations, sponsoring – all of these things would prove invaluable when I came to found Cinq Mondes. Two years later I was part of the TAG Heuer team, in charge of selling the company to LVMH.

The time had come to focus on a project of my own – particularly since by now my forays into Ayurvedic massage had led me to meet my future wife, Nathalie Bouchon. As a clinical psychologist passionate about holistic wellness, Nathalie would play a key role in setting up Cinq Mondes by arranging for research scientists to work in partnership alongside traditional healers.

So I left TAG Heuer and set off with Nathalie for an 18-month sabbatical to travel the world – or rather the "five worlds" of India, China, Japan, Siam and the Maghreb. I had

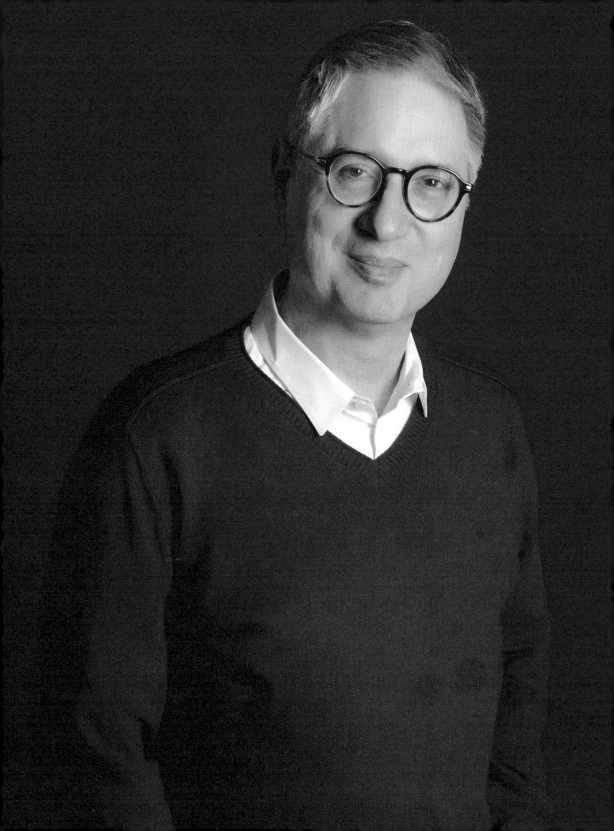

long ago realized that these "cinq mondes" were home to ancient rituals for wellness and beauty unrivaled anywhere else. We planned to find out more about those rituals, then modernize and adapt them to suit our western culture. Basically, we aimed to improve on tradition using the latest advances in eco-friendly cosmetology, with input from some of the greatest "noses" in the French perfume industry.

It was in the course of that world trip that I met Sri Sri Ravi Shankar, yoga guru, Indian spiritual leader and founder of one of the world's largest non-governmental organizations, The Art of Living. He taught us SudarShan Kriya: a breathing technique borrowed from meditation that works on mind-body balance. Through daily yoga practice and meditation, SudarShan Kriya breathing came to define our holistic approach to wellness and beauty, while also giving us the stamina and endurance to set up Cinq Mondes.

REALIZING
THE IMPOSSIBLE

The fact remained however that on our return to Paris in 2001 our Cinq Mondes project was no less daunting. Building a 5,300-square foot spa in the historic heart of Paris meant raising one million euros in funding – something that was well nigh impossible for the son of two retired English teachers. It meant selling our primary residence and putting every last dime into the business, raising the additional capital by borrowing money from the banks at two hundred per cent APR – the same banks that a month before meeting me thought "spa" referred to the French Société Protectrice des Animaux!

The company's survival in the first 18 months of trading seemed equally impossible. It depended on the spa being fully booked every day and on sales of Cinq Mondes cosmetics suddenly rocketing. Nothing less than a miracle, in other words.

In the end, it wasn't just one miracle but three.

" They didn't know it was impossible,
so they did it. "

MARK TWAIN

• Miracle Number One was the incredible media coverage surrounding the first Cinq Mondes spa: at least 1,000 press articles within a year of opening, including whole pages in *Vogue, Elle, Marie-Claire,* and two double-page spreads in *Air France Magazine* alone. That year we got even more attention from the French media than Clarins!

• As a direct consequence of Miracle Number One, six months after the opening of the first Cinq Mondes spa, we received a visit from Jacques Motet, owner of a five-star Relais & Chateaux Hotel in Grand Baie on the northwest coast of Mauritius. He turned up one morning waving a copy of the article in *Air France Magazine* and asked me to design a 1,500m2 (16,000 square feet) tropical-style spa for the grounds of his hotel – a franchise operating under the Cinq Mondes banner. It was the first in a series of 15 spas located in the finest hotels in Europe, Africa and the Middle East. Notable examples include the iconic Beau Rivage Palace in Lausanne and the Monte Carlo Bay in Monaco, both now featuring 1,500m2 Cinq Mondes spas.

• Miracle Number Three occurred shortly after opening thanks to Club Med CEO Henri Giscard d'Estaing. His strategy was to refocus on the holiday villages and attract upmarket vacationers, with the emphasis placed firmly on wellness, the body beautiful and self-care. As a champion of those values, I was called in to set up Cinq Mondes spas in La Palmeraie (Marrakech) and La Plantation d'Albion (Mauritius), two resorts that were repositioned in a new luxury category of so-called "5 Trident" villages. Each spa was run by a team of 30 people but operated as a subsidiary, not a franchise.

In 2001 when the spa business was virtually unheard of in France, nobody could ever have imagined the sheer speed of our growth. Through it all, I remained steadfastly optimistic, with an almost visceral belief in the future and a carefree outlook on life that however reckless, turned out to be my saving.

UNION OF MIND, BODY AND SPIRIT

In this book we will start by taking you on an 18-month journey of exploration across five different worlds with very particular traditions of wellness and beauty: the Cinq Mondes of India, China, Japan, Siam and Morocco. The beauty and wellness rituals that I discovered there opened my eyes and my mind to manual techniques of needle-free acupuncture that I called "dermapuncture;" and traditional medicines that inspired me to come up with my very own "skin nutrition program."

Though they originate from five different parts of the globe, all of these rituals have something important in common. The treatments they involve have been carefully rethought in line with the French-style art of living and state-of-the-art research in the French cosmetics industry (though still firmly based on ancient beauty rituals). Added to this, our range of aromatherapy products is the work of two of France's most respected noses, Olivia Giacobetti and Jean Pierre Béthouard.

Cinq Monde practitioners specialize in all of these treatments, making every one of our spas a modern-day temple of holistic wellness and beauty – places where the art of touch and healing combines with the power of plants to bring body, mind and skin into harmony, so reinforcing our conviction that, in the words of Paul Valéry, "The deepest part of a person is the skin."

As we shall see, the oldest systems of traditional medicine were quick to reflect on the essential connection between mind-body balance, health and younger skin at a cellular level – letting natural beauty show through.

First and foremost among those traditional systems is Ayurveda (from Sanskrit *veda* meaning knowledge, and *ayur* meaning life and longevity) which as we saw earlier is centered on the Abhyanga – traditional Indian massage with precious oils (neem, frankincense or sesame oil). Our doctor and scientific adviser Dr Gensham Marda studied the Abhyanga for 12 years and now holds a PhD in the subject (for which there is simply no equivalent in the West). Yoga (literally: "yoke" meaning the union of mind, body and soul) is another integral part of Ayurveda, the science of breathing providing the vital intermediary between psyche and soma.

HAPPINESS ON
A CELLULAR LEVEL

Indian and Ayurvedic traditions have so much to teach about the subtle connections between body and mind that we will use them to explore the art of pranayama (literally: vital life force) as taught by our spiritual master and yogi Sri Sri Ravi Shankar. Pranayama induces a meditative state that oxygenates every cell in our body, every neuron in our brain, thereby leading to deep relaxation and, with it, wellness, health and in a word, beauty.

The depth of pranayama holds enormous benefits for everyday living. So much so indeed that neuroscientists first in America then in Europe seized upon it as the basis for mindfulness and relaxation techniques that focus on the breath, so popularizing the concept of pranayama itself. Here again the subtle interplay between mind and body exerts an influence over the body and skin right down to the level of cellular

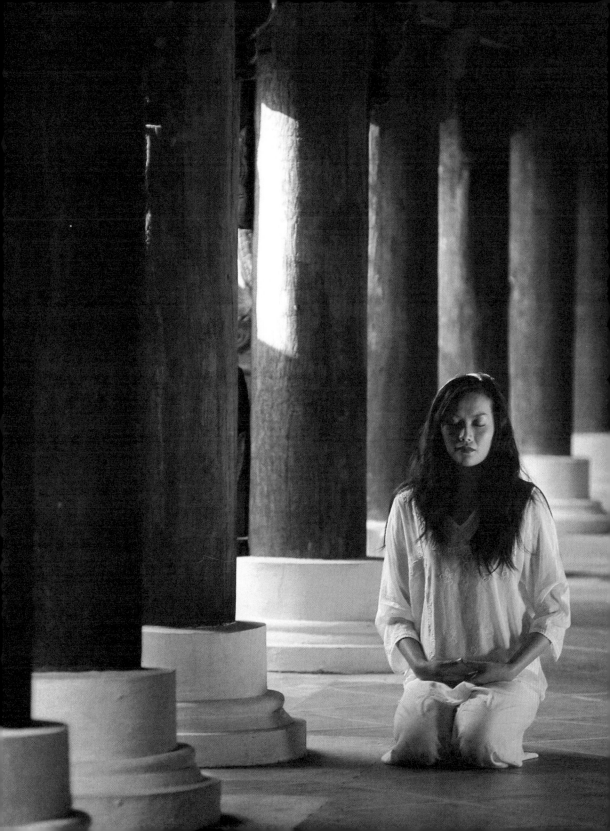

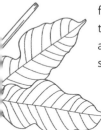

functioning. Hence the title of this book "Happiness within the skin," the skin being the ultimate reflection of the mind-body-spirit balance (or imbalance) and a holistic approach to wellness and beauty that is the key to "feeling comfortable in your own skin."

BRINGING TOGETHER
SCIENCE AND TRADITION

The thoughts and teachings in this book are also the fruit of our growth over the past 15 years. Working with specialists in dermo-cosmetology, Ayurvedic medicine, neuroscience and nutrition has taught us that health, beauty and nutrition are connected in more ways than one ...

This book will therefore look at those foods that nourish body and mind, and start by drawing a comparison between nutrition and cosmetics. Just as there are industrial foods and living foods, with all the differences in metabolic absorption imaginable, so there are industrial cosmetics and living cosmetics. On the one hand you have silicone or mineral-oil based products that leave an occlusive film on your skin like plastic wrap. On the other hand you have products made of natural oils and plant extracts that are readily absorbed by the skin.

With both types of products now on sale, consumers should be able to make an informed choice between the two.

Feeding the skin with essential fatty acids, such as Omega 3, 6 and 9, trace (oligo) elements, mineral salts and vitamins, helps to maintain cellular homeostasis (the equilibrium required for optimal functioning). Our modern lifestyle threatens that equilibrium due to what dermatologists call the "exposome:" the sum total of all the environmental factors in our lives. These factors can be external (sunlight, pollution, changes in temperature) or internal (cortisol for instance, a hormone associated with the oxidative stress that is a factor in premature skin aging). Improving our understanding of the exposome so as to prevent these imbalances is one of the core challenges facing cosmetics research over the next decade.

Our journey inside our skin cells will continue by exploring the cutaneous flora or microbiota: the billions of bacteria essential to the proper development, functioning and also the protection of cells. Because quite apart from the exposome, endocrine disruptors are another major problem facing public health authorities and the skincare industry.

Achieving and maintaining a subtle balance of forces is essential for homeostasis – a state that is to our skin cells what nirvana is to our consciousness.

This is why our research at Cinq Mondes focuses on exploring the benefits of dermapuncture combined with the guiding principles of our "skin nutrition program" – today and every day we are committed to making "happiness come from the skin!"

CINQ MŌNDES

élixir précieux®
éclat - radiance

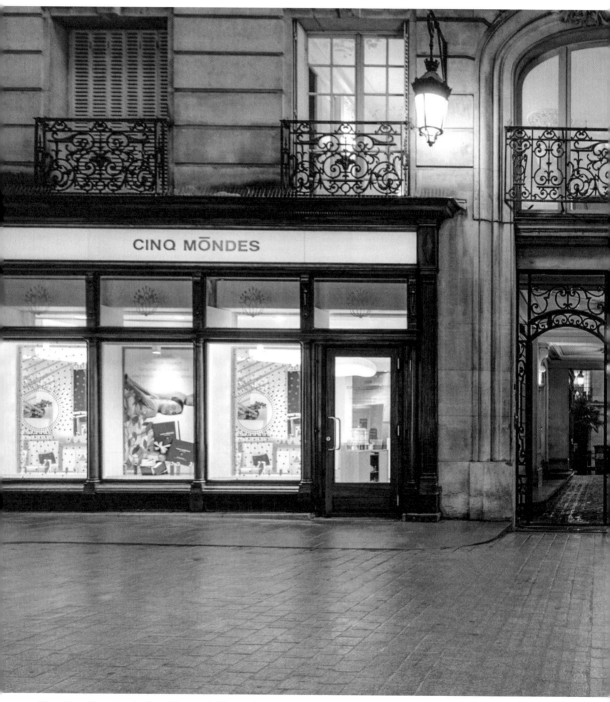

The oldest Cinq Mondes Spa, 6 Square de l'Opéra, Paris

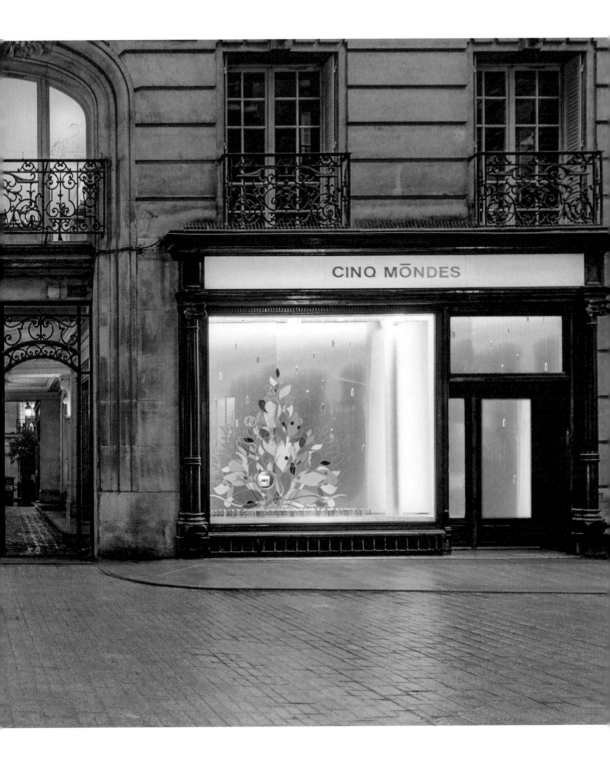

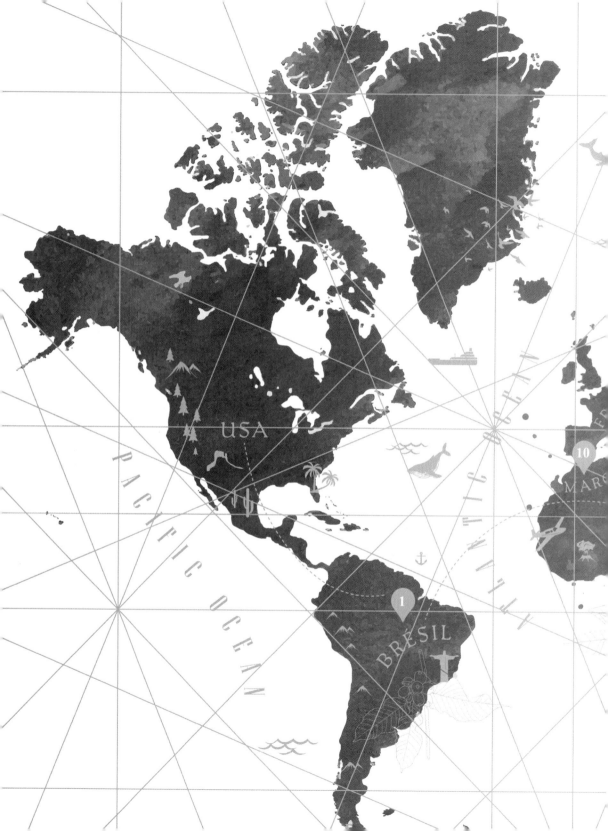

1

WHERE THE
CINQ MONDES SPAS
FIND THEIR
INSPIRATION

___

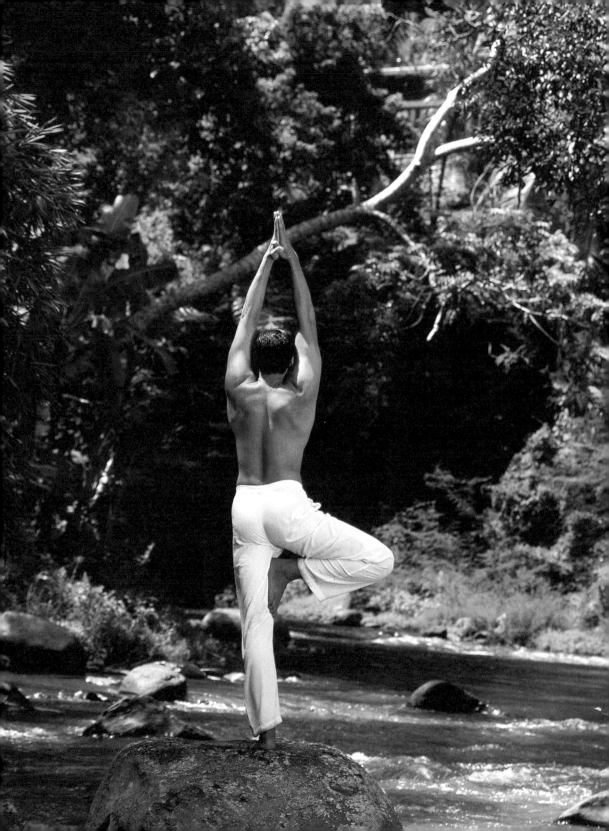

"Happiness comes from the skin" thus begins with foods that bring balance to the mind and body, thereby engendering a harmony that has an effect right down to the cells in the skin. This delicate balance between mind, body and spirit has been studied for centuries by the great traditional medicine systems of the Orient, which were the source of inspiration for American and Asian spas in the 1970s. They were also what led Nathalie and I to spend 18 months exploring the world from east to west, in search of the finest rituals of wellness and beauty on the planet. We dreamed of creating a French and European version of the spa – our very own temple of holistic wellness and beauty.

As it turned out, our timing couldn't have been better. Slowly but surely as we made our way around the world, we were handed the keys to an all-encompassing vision that embraces the physical, psychological, emotional and even spiritual dimensions of wellness and beauty.

Before we left, I picked five different "worlds" (India, Japan, China, Siam and Morocco) that met my three criteria: a written tradition of ancient wellness and beauty rituals; the existence of teachers and physicians associated with those traditions; and teachings that were still alive and kicking. These five regions were where we spent the most time, but we also checked out other spas along the way.

CANADA,
OR THE ASHRAM AS A MODEL OF "RURAL" INSPIRATION

Our world trip started with a stopover in Canada, first Montreal then Quebec. Few people are as passionate about nature and alternative therapies as the Canadians. We were there to attend a yoga retreat that was being organized by the Indian spiritual leader Sri Sri Ravi Shankar (whose teachings I had followed in Switzerland) at his ashram in Saint Mathieu du Parc. It was an invitation to silence, meditation and Ayurvedic healing, and of course to meet Sri Sri in person.

Those ten days were a powerful experience I shall never forget – a genuine initiation process that led me to renew the experience every year thereafter, either at the Bangalore ashram in India, or the Black Forest ashram in Bad Antogast, or another Art of Living Center founded by Sri Sri Ravi Shankar.

The infinitely subtle balance between body and mind

The daily routine at Saint Mathieu du Parc was a real revelation: up at 5am every morning; Shirodhara therapy at 6am (deep in meditation, you trickle warm sesame oil between your temples, letting it flow over your forehead); then, allowing for two vegetarian breaks in between, eight hours of yoga, meditation and pranayama, all practiced in complete silence – not a word was spoken for ten whole days.

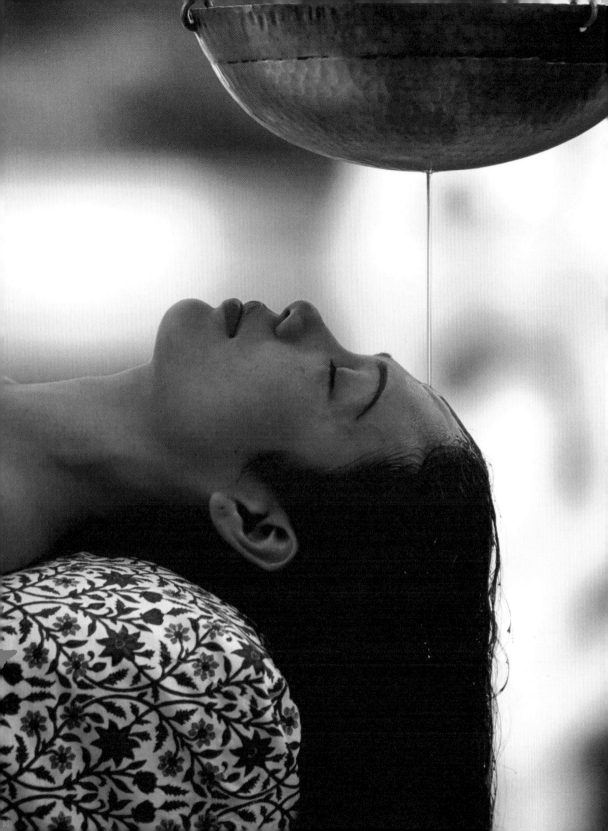

Just to complete the picture, this was the month of June and we had decided to camp – little knowing that we had pitched our tent on marshland and that it would rain hard for the duration of our stay. Every night we were invaded by clouds of mosquitoes – ferocious Canadian mosquitoes, known colloquially as *Maringoins*, five times the size of their European counterparts. Then there were the toads – a chorus of croaks that resounded all night with the percussive power of a djembe performance ... Indian sages say that being a bit tired helps you to meditate – just as well really, though in my case I didn't so much wake up tired as utterly exhausted.

SHIRODHARA TREATMENT

Shirodhara may not seem much to us Westerners, but it is in fact a highly refined art. In India they say it induces a sense of mind-body connection, a feeling that your whole being is in unison.

What is certain is that I made unimaginable progress in those ten days. Thanks to the Ayurvedic therapies, I could immediately almost touch that feeling of subtle balance that comes from greater body awareness as the body and mind gradually dissolve into one. The effect was a heightened mindfulness that was prolonged by early morning yoga and breathing practice, inducing a naturally meditative state that required no effort at all – a state you rarely get to achieve in a busy working life.

Silence or the end of "mental chatter"

My other great leap forward was the acceptance of silence – however unbearable it seemed in the beginning. For the first three days I was under constant bombardment from negative thoughts. "How did I end up in this quagmire?" "Why do we only ever get boiled vegetables to eat?" "When are those toads ever going to stop their cacophony?"

But eventually the yoga sessions brought feelings of peace, which were reinforced by Ayurvedic therapy. And every evening, there was the *darshan* with Sri Sri Ravi Shankar, whose words of wisdom brought answers to the questions we put to him in writing (only he was allowed to speak) about a whole range of subjects to do with Vedic traditions. After the darshan, we rounded off the day with traditional Indian chanting or *bhajans*.

THE DARSHAN

The darshan (literally "gaze" or "look") is a one-to-one or group discussion with a master. In the course of the darshan, the master gives advice and comments on sacred texts, so pupils can learn first-hand.

> *Silence is the goal of all answers. If an answer does not silence the mind, it is not a real answer. Only silence is complete. The goal of all words is to create silence.*
>
> Sri Sri Ravi Shankar

YOGA

Yoga is a branch of Ayurveda, based on poses (asanas) that work with the breath to bring every part of the body into proper balance and thereby free the spirit.

An oasis of inner peace

By the end of that initiation, I was committed to the idea of a spa focused on this essential connection between the mind, the body and the inner self. I had been made aware that the source of mental tranquility was healing therapy, yoga and meditation, and that breathing served as the intermediary between the body and the mind. I sensed that in the hyper-connected world for which we were headed, this oasis of inner peace would be precious beyond words to millions of city dwellers yearning to restore balance to their busy lives.

Obviously, my spas would not be ashrams where people would retreat into silence and lead a Spartan existence eating nothing but vegetarian food for ten days. But I now had a clear vision of what these spas would be – places dedicated to the pursuit of mental tranquility and the union of mind and body. From my experience at L'Oreal (cosmetics development) and TAG Heuer (luxury goods, spatial/shop/service design) I knew that what made my idea so original was its three-pronged approach: wholly natural therapies inspired by the great masters and physicians of the world's greatest cultures; a luxurious and elegant spa setting with the very highest standards of customer service; and a state-of-the-art cosmetics range endorsed by leading perfumers.

ASHRAM

Etymologically speaking, an Ashram is a place where there is no effort ("shram"). Maintain peace of mind and allow the energy to circulate within you effortlessly. This happens when we are at ease and in harmony with our environment. This is the meaning of Ashram: a place where we feel totally "at home."

The remainder of the journey would address all my questions, the answers fitting inside one another rather like Russian dolls ...

NORTH AMERICA:
THE POWER OF
AROMATIC IMMERSION

After Canada, we visited the east coast of the USA where I was impressed by the organization and "industrialization" of the local spas. It was in one of those stylish New York spas that I was greeted by a hostess dressed in black, who handed me a bottle of iced mineral water and yelled: "Your therapist is Sandy, Room 14, now!"

I decided then and there that my spas would take the opposite approach, offering a warm and gentle welcome more consistent with the art of hospitality French-style. I did however make a mental note of certain key operating principles ...

Our next stop was the West Coast, where a magical Japanese shiatsu experience awaited us in San Francisco: a feeling nothing short of bliss as the spa therapist pressed gently but firmly on specific points along the energy lines (the acupoints). Add to that a massage balm delicately scented with mint and cinnamon and you can see why I found the treatment so soothing ...

It was then that I decided to make aromatic immersion a key feature of Cinq Mondes therapy, smell and touch being our oldest, most primeval senses, operating beyond conscious thought to induce immediate relaxation.

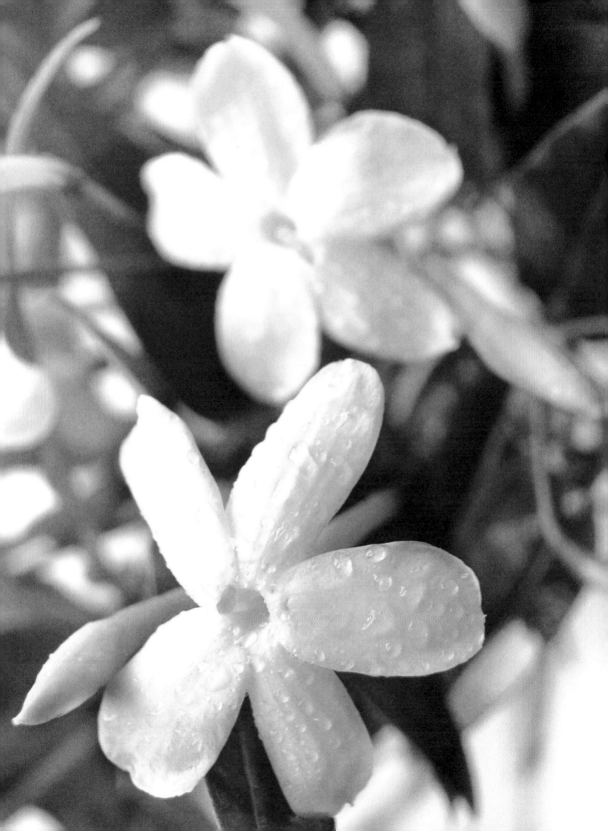

THE CONCEPT OF
NEEDLE-FREE ACUPUNCTURE
OR "DERMAPUNCTURE"

Back in Paris I would study shiatsu for two years under a Master of the Fédération Française de Shiatsu. I knew that shiatsu offered an approach that would underpin all of the techniques in the Cinq Mondes remit: "dermapuncture," a needle-free alternative to acupuncture, used in Ayurvedic medicine, Traditional Chinese Medicine (TCM) and traditional Japanese medicine (*shia-tsu* meaning "finger pressure" in Japanese).

Pressing on the acupoints boosts the flow of vital energy while also stimulating the lymphatic system, improving the tone, vitality and glow of the skin.

Thereafter each successive stopover in our five chosen destinations would shed new light on my thinking, bringing singular experiences that enriched the wellness techniques behind dermapuncture.

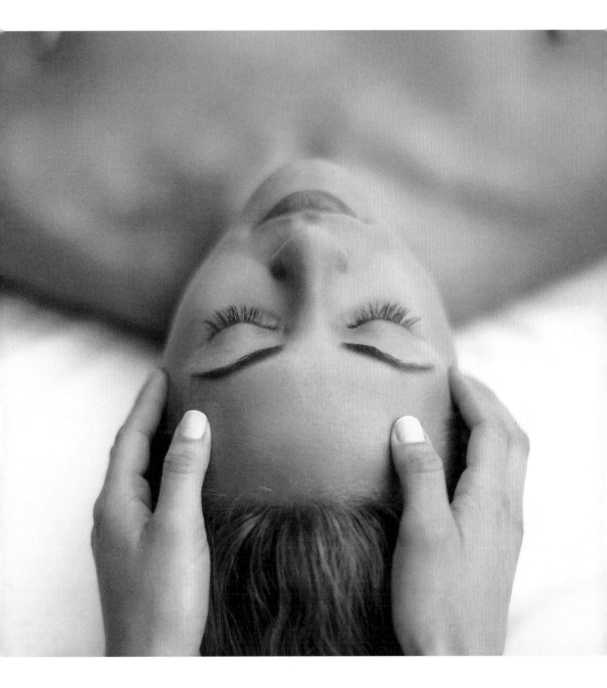

POLYNESIA
AND THE BENEFITS OF HERBAL MEDICINE AT ITS FINEST

In Polynesia we were welcomed by a yoga teacher friend of Nathalie's in Puna'auia, who let us stay in her yoga studio – a room with a bamboo parquet floor that looked out onto a tropical garden and the crystalline lagoon beyond. We spent two months there, practicing yoga and meeting native Polynesian healers, *tahuas*, who use massage as an aid to wellness. I also made solo visits to the national institute for agricultural research where I met an aging scientist with a most unusual story to tell ...

While working in his garden one day, he cut himself badly with one of his tools. Seizing the first fruit to hand, he opened it up and used the juice to relieve the pain. Imagine his surprise the following day to find that the wound was already healing. He had just discovered the extraordinary regenerative properties of the noni fruit (scientific name *Morinda citrifolia*), a plant native to Polynesia whose juice works at a cellular level and which is also drunk as a tonic to preserve health and prolong life.

As a firm believer in the power of plants, I threw myself into finding out everything there was to know about the local flora. One of the books I found particularly useful, highly recommended to fellow enthusiasts, was *L'Herbier* by Paul Pétard, a 300-page classic of its kind that documents every plant down to the last detail. And I decided to include noni and monoï oil in a "Baume de massage sublime", which was eventually launched eight years later. When looking to derive full benefit from rare plants, there are simply no shortcuts.

NONI

Morinda citrifolia or Noni is a tree in the Rubiaceae family that originally came from India, found mainly in tropical Pacific islands. It has been cultivated for more than 2,500 years in Polynesia where it is known for its medicinal benefits and considered sacred – hence its use in Polynesian initiation rituals.

THE THEORY
BEHIND "DERMAPUNCTURE"
AND MY
"SKIN DIETETICS PROGRAM"

Henceforth, wherever we traveled, I sought to develop a connection between what I called "dermapuncture" – stimulating key energy points throughout the body and in the skin tissue – and the use of the most powerful plant-based active ingredients in the local pharmacopeia. By also feeding the skin with nutrients that stimulate cell metabolism, I aimed to arrive at the "ultimate skin nutrition program."

So I spent my time partly scouring villages, pharmacies and tribal settlements for ancient beauty secrets and active plant extracts; and partly being tutored in massage therapy by traditional teachers and healers. In Thailand for instance, I later spent five months in Chiang Mai attending daily classes in traditional *Nuad Boran* massage, eventually completing every level from One to Six (the so-called "teacher's level").

The next stage, in Japan, would yield major discoveries on both fronts.

JAPAN
AND THE ART OF KOBIDO

In Kyoto we were introduced to the art of Kobido: an ancient form of facial massage that falls under the umbrella of Shiatsu therapy. Kobido is a wonderfully complex technique, combining 50 movements that produce a natural lifting effect using only the fingertips to apply pressure to specific points on the face. For 90 minutes, deft fingers gently pinch, knead and stroke the skin, a feeling like being caressed by butterfly wings. Kobido is a moment beyond time that leaves you deliciously relaxed, with your complexion smoother, firmer and plumper. The etymology of the word reveals its inspiration: *ko* means "ancient", *bi* means beauty and *do* means "way". Since it was first introduced to France, 1,000 Cinq Mondes partner spas in 36 countries have named Kobido as one of the most effective anti-aging techniques for the skin and face.

KOBIDO

Kobido facial massage uses three main techniques:

– shiatsu (finger pressure massage) to stimulate energy points that boost skin vitality;

– skin-rolling to tone facial muscles;

– lifting movements to tighten and soften the expression and smooth out any lines.

The power of traditional medicine

Also in Kyoto, my forays into Japanese traditional medicine (formulae grouped together over two thousand years to form a branch of medicine called the *Kampo*) gave me the idea for the essential corollary to Kobido: a skincare product that when applied in the course of the massage, would help to regenerate skin cells. Harnessing the formidable antioxidant powers of shiso (*Perilla frutescens*) and the lotus flower (*Sophora japonica*), I later developed a recipe for an anti-aging cream – Crème Précieuse© Cinq Mondes – that included the patented active ingredients of avena

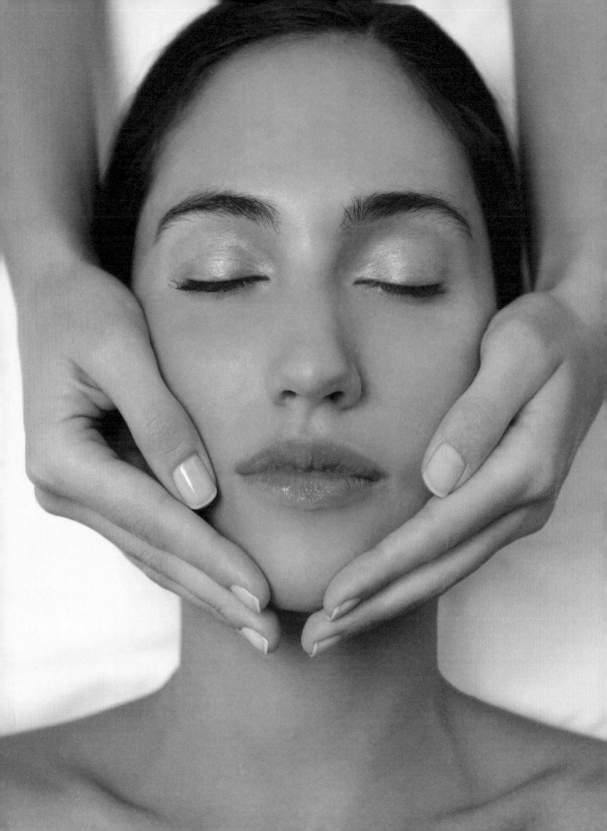

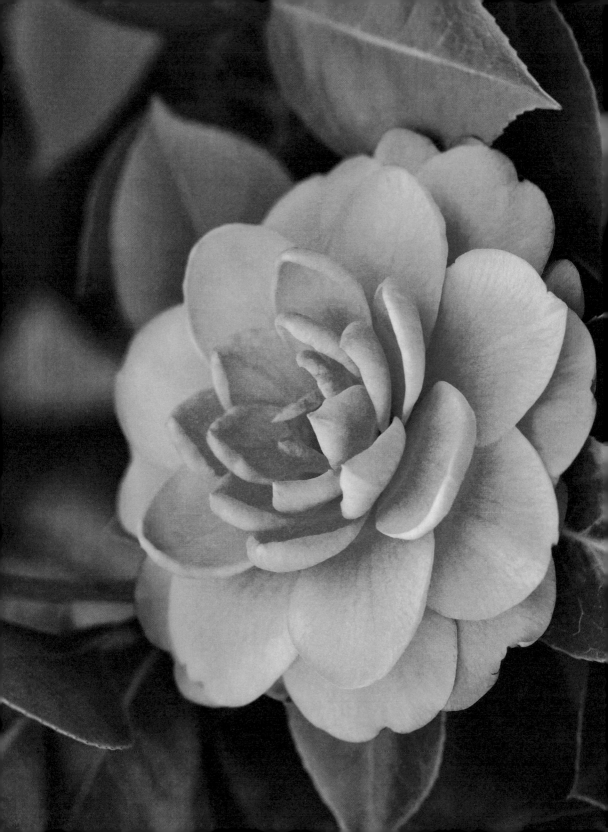

sativa and arbutin … I also discovered the exceptional qualities of camellia oil: a rich source of the essential fatty acids Omega 3, 6 and 9, plus nutrients with a structural and chemical affinity for the skin, most notably the lipids within our famous acid mantle. This allowed me to come up with groundbreaking innovations in anti-aging skincare.

I did of course wonder at the time why so many skincare creams were essentially silicone or mineral-oil based, with no affinity whatsoever with the skin, and an effect that basically comes down to covering the skin in plastic to hide any imperfections – flattering certainly, but it prevents the skin from breathing. The answer, as I realized a few months later back in Paris, is quite simple. As petroleum byproducts, silicones are almost ten times cheaper than plant-based alternatives: nine euros a kilo compared to 150 euros for oils with miraculous regenerative properties like camellia, tamanu and kemiri oil.

The choice was mine, and as you might guess I chose the more expensive option. Rare and precious oils inspire the formulas of all Cinq Mondes cosmetics, most notably the "élixirs précieux", which are made from one hundred percent essential oils. The action exerted by these unique substances sheds light on the concept of assimilation – a key concept in terms of internal nutrition, but also topical nutrition or what I prefer to call "skin nutrition."

CAMELIA SINENSIS

Camellia Sinensis and its characteristic flowers, also known as green tea, comes from a species of shrub in the family Theaceae known for its remarkable antioxidant and skin protection properties.

The Japanese "Ofuro" or bath: more than just hygiene, a time for contemplation

Our trip to Japan would not have been complete without a Japanese bath – a core wellness therapy that I had in fact discovered many years earlier.

The Japanese bathing ritual (because it is definitely a ritual) is not so much about washing as about relaxing, meditating and nourishing the body and soul. Japan is the only country in the world where you can be invited to soak in an *ofuro* tub before dinner (depending of course on your host and the venue in question). A surprising custom certainly, but for me highly inspirational too. So much so that the bathtub we designed for the Cinq Mondes – a masterpiece of cabinetmaking – has become emblematic of our spas. As if the ritual were not already sufficiently refined, we go a step further by offering a flower petal bath combined with customized aromatherapy and a neck and shoulder massage ...

THE OfURO BATH

The name Ofuro denotes a bathtub in unfinished natural wood, typically with a lid that helps keep the water warm (at least 40°C/104°F). The idea is to wash beforehand then unwind in the bath, escaping the everyday as you lose yourself in quiet contemplation of the landscape or an inspiring object. Once your spirit is recharged, invigorated by its flight to other realms, you are ready to return to normal activity (dinner, massage, work ...).

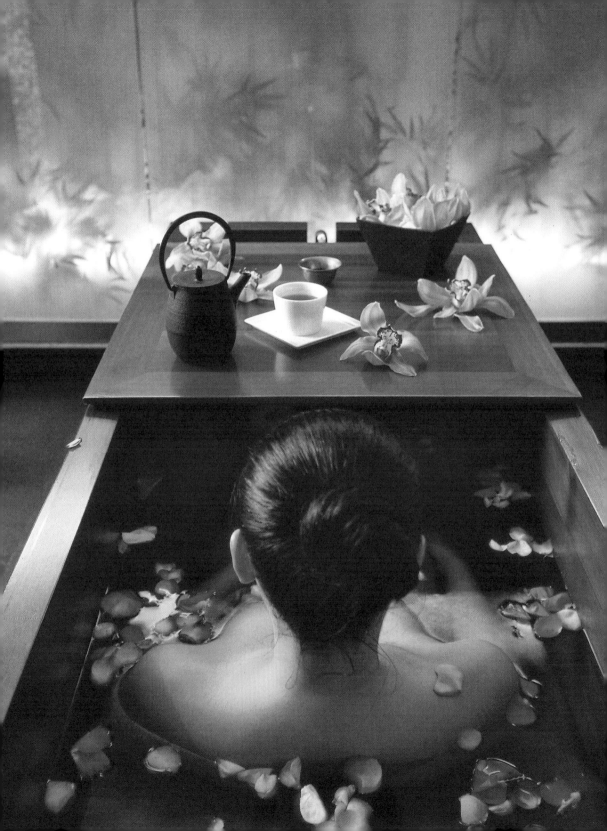

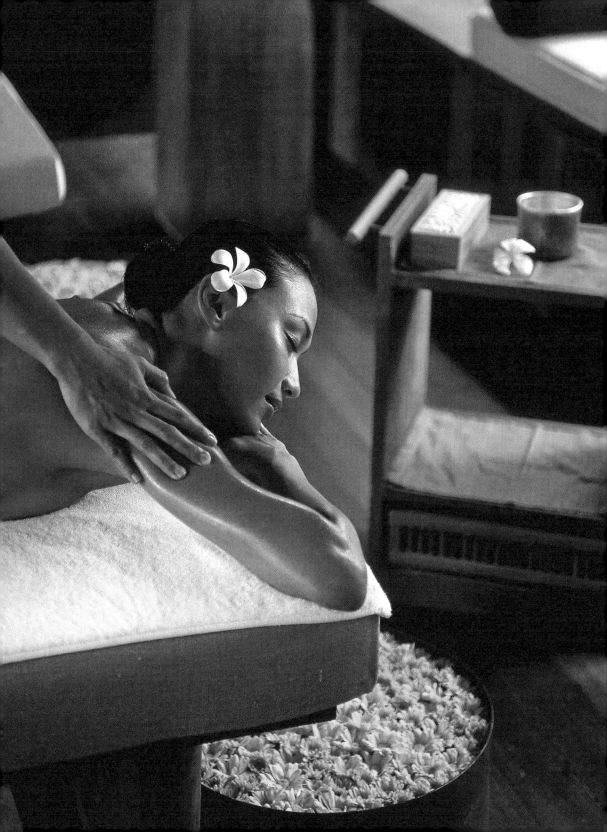

BALI,
OR THE POWER
OF FLOWERS AND FRUITS

For me the most surprising thing about our world training and study tour was the realization that the ancient beauty secrets I discovered all depended on properties that science and cosmetics research could understand and explain to the modern consumer. Balinese traditional medicine was a case in point ...

The skin of a Balinese princess ...

Ubud, in the center of the island of Bali, is home to an ancient beauty ritual dating back to the 16th century that has survived to this day among young women of the local nobility. It consists of rubbing a mixture of papaya flesh and crushed rice on the skin to remove dead cells and restore radiance to the complexion – what we now call a body scrub.

Five centuries later we know that the papaya enzyme papain has a strong "kerato-lytic" action, meaning that it breaks down intercellular bonds so helping to remove dead skin cells and impurities. It imparts an incomparable glow to the skin, as if a veil of dullness has been lifted to let the radiance show through. So it is that the effects discovered by ancient Balinese herbalists, based solely on empirical observation, can now be explained by modern science.

On my return to Paris I set to work adapting these recipes, adding new active ingredients aimed at enhancing their efficacy and feel, with no loss of their original qualities. Crushed rice for example has the disadvantage of dissolving in modern cosmetics formulas and losing its exfoliating effect. So I replaced it in our "Purée de Papaye" with diatomaceous earth and tiny grains of marine minerals (no more than 50 microns in diameter), so producing a softer but equally efficient body scrub with the same enzymatic and mechanical activity as its traditional Balinese counterpart. Suitable for even the most sensitive skin, our "Purée de Papaye" also includes a plant-based surfactant that, unlike its Balinese predecessor, makes it easy to remove after application. On contact with water it produces a light lather like mild soap that simply washes off – making it perfect for people who want to exfoliate in the shower.

It is fascinating work to retrace the origins of ancient beauty recipes then modernize them in accordance with the latest cosmetics technology. What is more it makes it possible to offer an infinitely more natural approach to beauty than petrochemical beauty – an approach that shows infinitely more respect for the skin and the environment.

PASSION FRUIT

Passion fruit, also known as granadilla, is a small tropical berry about the size of an egg. It is commonly added to cosmetics (scrubs and moisturizers) for its excellent healing and antioxidant properties – as a rich source of beta-carotene it stimulates melanin production giving you a healthy glow!

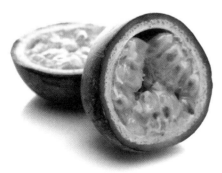

The beauty secrets of Balinese dancers

Exchanging ideas with Balinese herbalists and the local keepers of age-old traditions also taught me how Balinese stage actresses once removed their heavy make-up (the equivalent of modern waterproof make-up). They applied a mixture of mango butter and passion fruit oil, which quite literally dissolved the pigments and rid the skin of any residue. This was used in conjunction with slightly acidic tropical flowers for an even more lustrous complexion.

On my return to Paris I shut myself away in my laboratory to work on a make-up remover of my own: "Pâte de Fleurs", an improved version of the ancient Balinese recipe, with the same qualities but kinder to the skin thanks to an emulsifier that eliminates every last trace of make-up. Fifteen years later, that modern take on an ancient beauty recipe is available in 36 countries and ranks as one of Cinq Mondes' best-selling products – proving that an alliance of tradition, modernity and nature at its purest can inspire industrially produced cosmetics and revolutionize conventional wisdom.

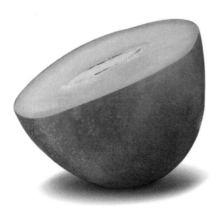

MANGO BUTTER

The Mango tree is native to southern Asia, especially India and Burma, and confined to tropical countries. The flesh of the mango fruit is eaten raw and used in cooking, but the stone contains kernels that are extracted to make mango butter. Produced exclusively from plant-based ingredients, mango butter is an excellent moisturizing agent, recommended for skin and hair alike.

PARIS
AND THE REALIZATION
OF A VISION

It is still a thrill to design spas with 1,000, 2,000 or 3,000 square meters of space (from 11,000 to 32,000 square feet) that is dedicated to holistic wellness – sumptuous settings for wellness and beauty rituals gleaned from the far corners of the globe. But for me that 18-month voyage of discovery was just a beginning. Every year since the creation of Cinq Mondes, I take off for another two months of exploration in search of time-honored beauty rituals that can be adapted and improved to suit modern lifestyles. These core principles never change.

The challenge is ever to create the ideal conditions for optimal wellness, to nourish the body, mind and skin. Thanks to modern science, we now know more than ever before about the absorption of topically applied substances through the skin. In Part 2 of this book we will see just how far our scientific knowledge of the skin absorption process has progressed.

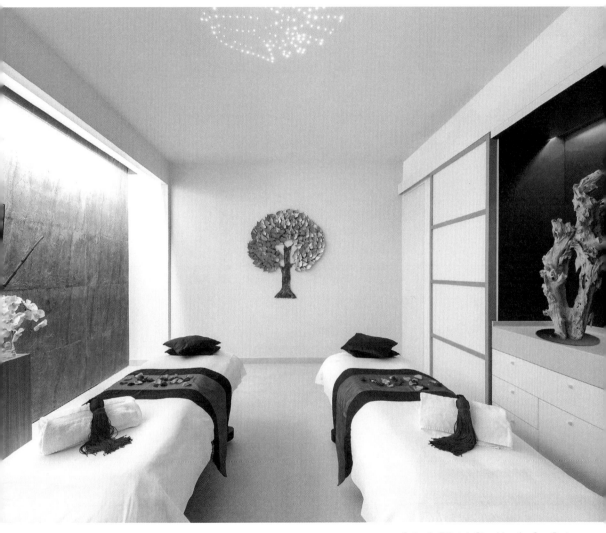

Suite de Félicité, Cinq Mondes Spa, Paris

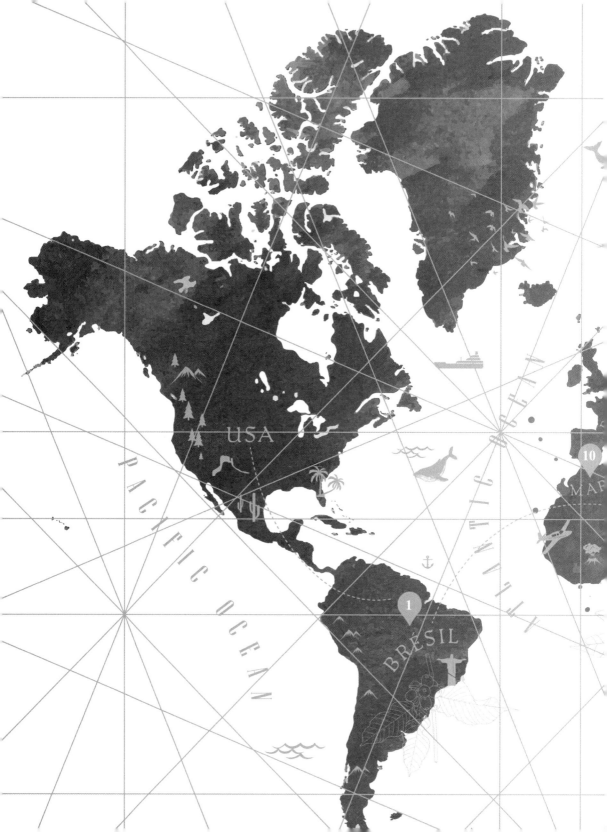

2

THE TIME-HONORED
SYSTEM OF AYURVEDA

___

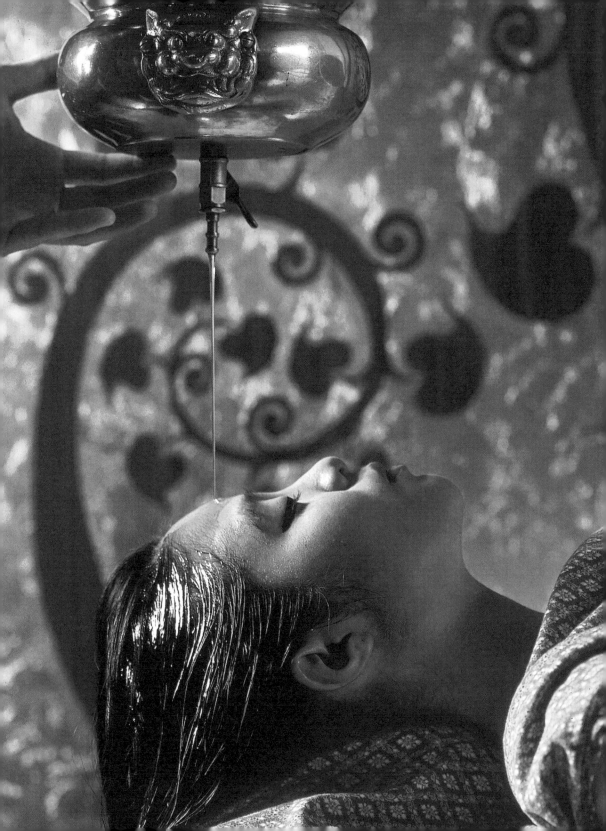

"Take care of your body so that your soul may wish to inhabit it."

SANSKRIT PROVERB

As we have seen, before founding Cinq Mondes I traveled the world for more than a year in search of traditional medicines and herbal remedies. Ayurveda obviously came top of the list, representing a system of medicine that met three of the criteria we had set for ourselves: a well-documented literary tradition; teachers and masters who were prepared to share their knowledge with Westerners; and skills that were still practiced today.

Better still, by emphasizing the prevention of illness, Ayurveda represents a total way of life that centers on herbal medicines, purifying treatments such as fasting and expert massage.

AYURVEDA:
A PHILOSOPHY
AND A WAY OF LIFE

Prior to leaving France, I attended classes in Ayurvedic massage in Paris that taught me the roots of the philosophy behind the Ayurvedic way of life. Literally, Ayurveda means science of longevity (from *ayur*, life or longevity, and *veda*, science or knowledge). It gave birth to a system of holistic medicine that survives to this day in India, but essentially stands for an all-embracing vision of life that sees balance as the path to happiness. Hence the Sanskrit word for healthy: *swastha* or "self-abiding" (from *swa*, own, self and *stha*, stable, steady). The concept of health is thus defined as an ideal state of equilibrium, of centered happiness. Ill health on the other hand, disrupts that equanimity, makes you feel out of control and at odds with yourself. The expression "being out of sorts" puts it nicely.

In the beginning: the benefits of massage

Thanks to my partner Nathalie, I had also made an amazing scientific discovery. In the course of her work as a clinical psychologist, Nathalie had attended a course in the neonatal intensive care unit of the Pontoise Hospital in the Paris area, where she had observed first-hand the effects of massage on premature infants. While some of the babies were simply placed in incubators others also received daily massage therapy – with a concomitant 50 per cent decrease in the infant mortality rate.

The benefits of the massage were thus systemic, acting on the body-mind connection, and not confined to specific muscles or inducing a state of wellbeing. Massage works via the skin, which is the body's largest organ, connected to all the other organs including the brain by way of infinite interconnections, and via trillions of neurotransmitters. It stimulates the release of hormones vital to life, most notably dopamine, serotonin and endorphins. In this way, massage works the organs on all levels – physically, emotionally and even spiritually. Far more than a mere adjunct to physiotherapy, massage is a treatment in its own right.

This is very much the message conveyed by Ayurveda, a traditional medicine system dating back more than five thousand years.

The origins of Ayurveda

Among the great traditions that have contributed so much to mankind, those origi-nating on the Indian sub-continent date back further than most. In the Valley of the Indus, in present-day northwest India, archaeologists have discovered evidence of an advanced civilization that can be traced back to the fourth or third millennium BC. The evidence includes vegetative remains found at the sites of Mohenjo-Daro and Harappa that testify to the use of medicinal plants, suggesting a culture with a particular focus on health and hygiene. Some of these plants are still used to make Western drugs today. Also at these sites are numerous vestiges of private and public baths including, most especially, early wastewater recycling systems.

Ayurveda is known to have been practiced there since time immemorial. The other Vedas ("Books of Knowledge", the foremost sacred texts in Hinduism), particularly Arthada-Veda (3000 BC), are filled with anatomical descriptions and descriptions of illnesses and how to treat them. But the two foundational Ayurvedic texts that have survived from ancient India – the *Charaka-Samhita* and the *Susruta-Samhita* – show just how much these civilizations knew about medicine thanks to the support of Buddhist rulers who upheld medical practices in order to demonstrate their compas-sion for all living beings.

Thereafter, Ayurvedic medicine evolved over time, most notably by incorporating the precepts of the Unani Greco-Arab medicine system that was introduced to India by the Islamic invaders. It was then banned under British rule in an effort to stamp out a system that the Raj considered worthless, only regaining its former status when India became independent.

The basis of Ayurvedic medicine is that living well is only possible when the body and mind are in harmony.

In search of a master

Varkala is a fishing village in Kerala, perched at the top of small cliffs where sacred cows graze peacefully in the shade of coconut trees. While we were staying there, we heard from some fellow travelers that a certain Doctor Babu Joseph was coming to his home town of Cochin, slightly further north up the coast, to teach Westerners the art of Abhyanga: Ayurvedic self-massage, based on harmonizing the vital functions and allowing the energy to flow. We arranged to meet him the following Monday ... and waited until Wednesday for him to arrive!

His teachings were fascinating but we decided not to continue because what we really needed was a scientific partner who met our three criteria: a perfect command of English; a good working knowledge of Europe (ideally a medical doctor who travelled there regularly); and a research-based approach to Ayurvedic therapy.

As a student of Ayurvedic massage therapy in Paris, my teachers had told me about a young doctor and scientist in Ayurvedic research, Doctor Ghanashyam Marda, who ran a clinic in Pune, north of Bombay. We went to visit him there and were instantly taken by his passion for communication and heartfelt commitment to reviving an ancient system of medicine that had for too long remained in the shadow of Western allopathic medicine following decades of British colonialism.

Dr Marda was the perfect embodiment of the revival and spread of Ayurvedic practices in India but also in Europe. Better still, he actually had a PhD in Ayurveda, having spent 12 years at university, the while writing his doctoral thesis on "The effects of

> " *When you arrive at the door of a spiritual Master, endless searching ends and fulfillment begins.* "
>
> SRI SRI RAVI SHANKAR

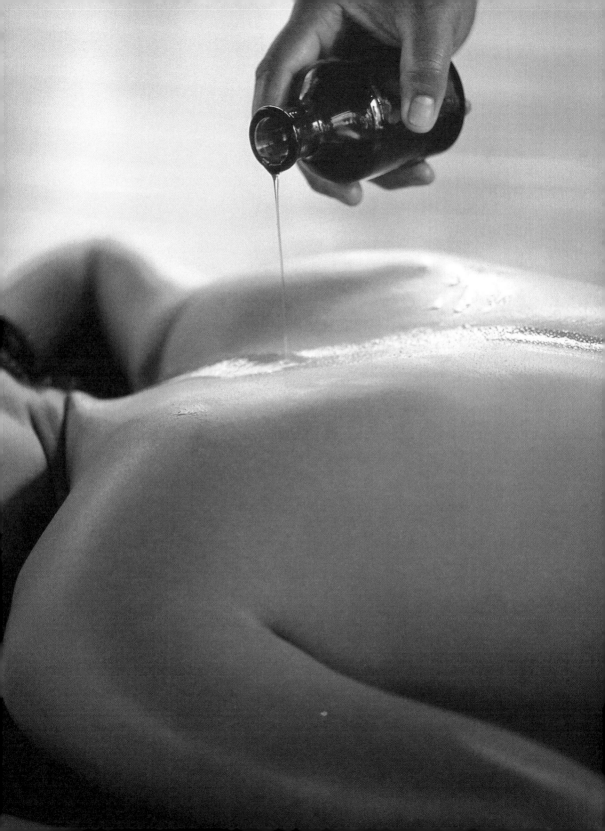

massage on psychosomatic illness." An unthinkable subject in France where doctors have always dismissed massage – not to mention the benefits of preventive health care, exercise, nutrition and sleep – and concentrated solely on fixing illnesses after they occur. But then again, massage in France is a job for *masseurs kinésithérapeutes* (masseur physiotherapists), not for doctors with 12 years of schooling behind them. And your typical *masseur kinésithérapeute* knows a lot more about physiotherapy than massage – which is harder work for less money.

For Dr Ghanashyam Marda, Ayurveda offered a fascinating approach to a medical practice based on careful observation of the subtle balances between the body and the spirit but also, of course, the skin as a vital organ of the human body. A medical practice, what is more, whose primary goal is not so much to treat illness as to prevent people from becoming sick in the first place. This it does by providing advice on diet and healthy living aimed at maintaining a state of physical and emotional wellbeing – a sense of plenitude and "happiness" that begins at the cellular level. In short a "happiness that comes from the skin."

Such was the essence of his teachings while we were staying at his clinic in Pune and on each of his quarterly, ten-day visits to Europe for 15 years thereafter.

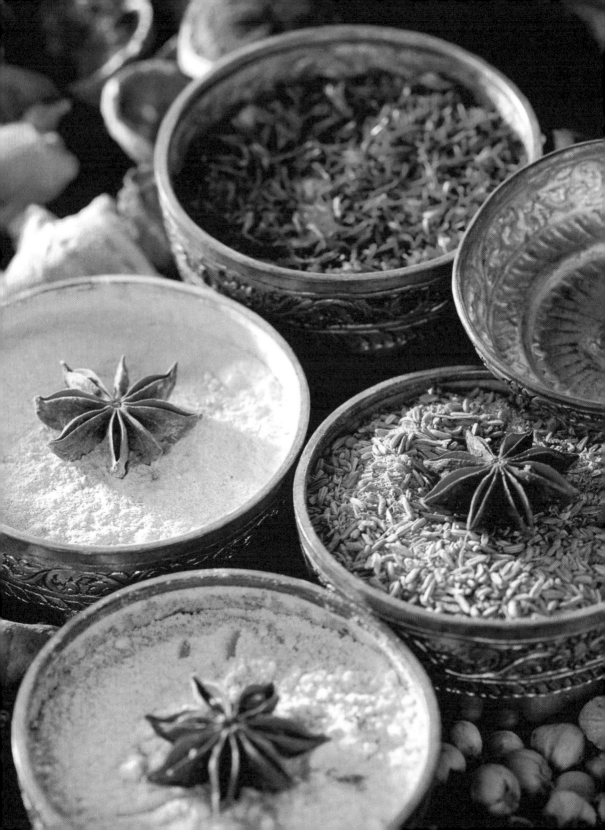

AYURVEDA OR THE ANCIENT
INDIAN ART OF WELLBEING

by Dr Ghanashyam Marda,
doctor of Ayurvedic medicine

Dr Marda practices Ayurvedic medicine in his clinic near Mumbai and is the Director of the Ayurveda Foundation, an association of Ayurvedic doctors whose mission is to promote traditional medicine in India. Dr Marda teaches and lectures in India and Europe: he is a senior lecturer at the College of Ayurveda, Middlesex University, London; and at Ayurveda research centers in Germany, Italy, Portugal, Denmark and Romania. He is committed to ongoing research into the benefits of massage and Ayurvedic remedies and to Panchakarma as a treatment for Type 2 diabetes, psychosomatic disorders and heart disease. He also works as a consultant to Cinq Monde spas in the field of Indian healing traditions.

"Modern life becomes increasingly stressful. We all suffer from information overload and this gradually wears us down mentally and physically. So each of us must find concrete ways to relieve stress on a daily basis.

For Ayurveda, the traditional Indian medicine system, health means more than just the absence of illness. The primary goal of Ayurveda is to help people lead whole and happy lives through physical and mental wellbeing.

In Ayurvedic culture, the word for health is swastha, from swa "inner" and stha "to stay". Health in India thus refers to whole-person wellbeing, the inner self radiating outward, not just physical wellbeing.

Most of the time when we are tired, stressed and tense, our whole being becomes unbalanced and off-center. Ayurveda offers us many ways to restore harmony to body and mind and so return to a state of balance.

According to Ayurvedic teaching, there are three principle energies in the body, or doshas. These three doshas are the manifestations of elemental forces in the physical body. Vata dosha is formed by the interaction of space and air. Pitta dosha embodies qualities similar to fire. Kapha dosha is formed by the interactions of water and earth.

All of the processes in the physical body are governed by the balance of doshas. One dosha tends to be dominant in any individual, giving them a specific dosha constitution. Each dosha type has its particular strengths and weaknesses. Perfect health is achieved when these three principle energies are in balance.

Massage is central to Ayurveda, a form of treatment that maintains balanced health and prevents the majority of imbalances. For best results, massage employs plant oils containing active ingredients that nourish and revitalize. These oils are used throughout the massage and correspond to the particular needs of the different dosha types inside and out. In India the choice of oil is in the hands of the physician and also depends on the season and the environment."[1]

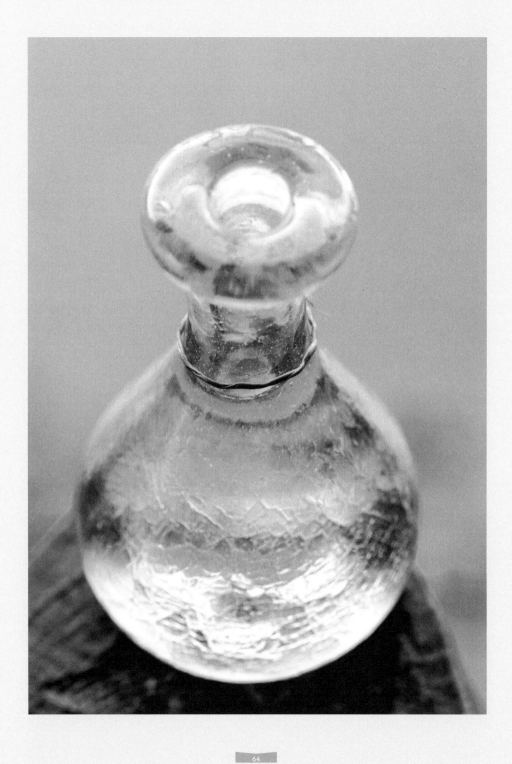

THE PRINCIPLES
OF AYURVEDA

According to Ayurveda, the universe or macrocosm is composed of five basic physical elements: space, air, fire, water and earth. These in turn give rise to three immaterial forces or energies called the doshas. The human microcosm is simply the macrocosm in miniature, born of the same five elements and three doshas. Balancing the doshas, which each has its own strengths and weaknesses, is the lynchpin of Ayurvedic physiology, essential to bring the body into balance.

The three doshas

In Ayurveda, everything in the universe is thus made up of the same "stuff", which shapes our individual nature: the five elements of air, fire, water, earth and space (or the ether). These five elements combine with each other to form three doshas or "constitutional" types. Our body balance depends on working in harmony with these doshas, which coexist in every human being though one is usually dominant.

Dosha in Sanskrit means "that which changes." The three doshas combine with each other in ever changing patterns of energy, affecting our mood, emotions, physical constitution and qualities.

- **Vata Dosha is comprised of the elements air and ether, related to movement and kinetic energy;**

- **Pitta Dosha is comprised of the elements fire and water, related to metabolism and transformation;**

- **Kapha Dosha is comprised of the elements water and earth, related to preservation and the energy of cohesion.**

As these three forces constantly move in and out of balance, they define our individual strengths and weaknesses. Every personality is defined by the dominance or conspicuous lack of one particular dosha. So understanding your dosha is essential for a balanced life – when it is out of sync we typically fall sick or feel "off". Restoring harmony depends on rebalancing these three energetic forces, which have a direct impact on our health, beauty and powers of rejuvenation.

The Ayurvedic physician therefore provides us with guidelines for living based on an analysis of the doshas present. These guidelines cover every aspect of our life – nutrition, physical activity, medicines and much more besides. Foods for example are grouped according to their characteristics (sour, acid, spicy, sweet, salty or astringent) and their influence on the dosha. Vata individuals are naturally drawn to salty, acid and sweet tastes; Pitta individuals to sweet, sour and astringent tastes; and Kapha individuals to spicy/sour tastes and cooked food.

But before we look at which foods are best suited to rebalance specific body-mind constitutions, let us first look at the different characteristics of these three doshas.

Vata, dosha of Movement

Vata is the energy of movement, related to vitality and rhythm in general. Vata individuals are enthusiastic, impulsive, communicative, idealistic, creative and passionate. Vata is known for having the quality of wind and space at its heart – dry, light, cold, mobile, etc. In the body, Vata manifests as breathing, the nervous system, the movement of food through the digestive tract and locomotion. In the mind, Vata governs the senses and reflex actions such as sneezing.

When Vata is in balance, it coordinates our bodily processes and keeps them functioning smoothly. Vata helps with good sleep and normal hormonal activity.

Signs of imbalance due to excess Vata include: skin dryness, excess nervous energy, poor sleep, bloating, trembling, uncoordinated limb movements and sometimes apathy and depression.

How to balance Vata: this usually requires changing your lifestyle and diet and taking the appropriate herbal remedies. For instance:

- **Perform breathing exercises for centering and grounding to combat racing thoughts and anxiety.**

- **Do less, slow down, avoid sensory stimulation of all kinds, go to bed early.**

- **Apply essential oils for dry skin – those rich in fatty acids such as sesame oil and wheat germ oil.**

- **Switch to a diet of mild-tasting foods: rich, moist, hot dishes, nothing too sweet, salty or sour. Raw onions and peppers for instance, aggravate Vata. Eat well in the morning then little and often throughout the day. Avoid cold drinks, which exacerbate anxiety disorders – stick to herb teas.**

- **Go for herbal remedies known for their soothing properties: chamomile, licorice, cinnamon, verbena, melissa, burdock and passion flower. Also plants that promote digestion: fennel, ginger, cardamom, basil, thyme, mint and rosemary.**

Pitta, the dosha of Transformation

Pitta is the energy of transformation, related to heat, cooking, the conversion of food to energy, emotions, metabolism, appetite and thirst. Pitta is formed from the interaction of fire and water, characterized by lightness, speed and fluidity. It manifests as courage, ambition, willpower and desire.

Signs of imbalance due to excess Pitta include: intense hunger and thirst, burning sensations and inflammation, plus feelings of impatience, aggression, anger and a generally bossy attitude.

How to balance Pitta:

- **Spend time in the great outdoors (in a forest or by a river) enjoying the fresh air and the light. The most simple joys and pleasures can bring the most happiness, helping to calm overheated emotions and the negative feelings caused by excess Pitta.**

- **Apply soothing essential oils to the skin that help heal and regenerate the tissues and prevent acidity and irritation. Neem oil is ideal, derived from the fruits and seeds of a tree with so many healing benefits that in India they call it the "village pharmacy."**

- **Stick to low-fat foods, preferably fresh, raw food with a sweet/sour/astringent taste, but eaten in sufficient quantities to satisfy the Pitta appetite. Avoid anything too acidic – peppers, citrus, mangoes, pineapple, tomatoes – and eat plenty of alkaline-producing foods such as parsley, fresh coriander and lettuce.**

- **Go for herbal remedies known for their antacid and detoxifying properties – horsetail, dandelion and nettle – plus remedies that support liver and kidney function.**

Kapha, the dosha of Protection

Kapha is the energy of protection, related to stability, order, structure, softness, physical and mental strength, stamina and perseverance. Kapha is formed from the interaction of earth and water, characterized by cold, heaviness, steadiness, slowness and sensuality. It promotes anabolism, warding off sickness and maintaining immunity.

Signs of imbalance due to excess Kapha include: fatigue, asthenia, emotional and intellectual dullness, heavy legs, sadness or melancholia, weight gain and water retention.

How to rebalance Kapha:

- **However difficult, devote time to physical exercise and outdoor activities. Exposure to sunlight is particularly effective to help lift the spirits and shake off heaviness and bad habits. Train your body to sleep less. Get outside and enjoy Nature. Move more – take up sport, travel. Staying active may be hard but it's worth the effort.**

- **Apply warming essential oils to the skin that stimulate the epidermis: frankincense oil for instance, mixed with vanilla and cardamom.**

- **Switch to a diet of low-fat foods, preferably light meals, served hot and seasoned with spices and condiments that stimulate the digestive fire. Stick to reasonable portions and avoid anything too heavy – no fried foods, patisserie or richly sauced dishes. Favor green vegetables such as salads, chicory and radishes plus herbs such as parsley.**

- **Go for warming, invigorating herbal remedies – ginger, hibiscus, ginseng, mustard, chili – plus remedies that support the digestion such as cardamom, ginger, pepper, vanilla and rosemary.**

Where more in-depth treatment is required, only a seasoned Ayurvedic practitio-ner is qualified to diagnose the imbalances and prescribe the appropriate curative approach. But developing self-awareness and intuition helps us to understand our basic constitution and adapt accordingly – adjusting our lifestyle to maintain a deli-cate balance of energies. For instance, people with a tendency to excess Vata should practice sports that ground the body and unclutter the mind. Kapha types prone to asthenia should seek out the sun; and excitable Pitta types should use breathing exercises to reduce irritability.

AYURVEDA
IN SCHOOL

In India school-teachers trained in Ayurveda are able to distinguish between pupils based on their particular dosha type – Vata, Pitta or Kapha – and adapt their teaching accordingly. Kapha types need more physical exercise (amongst other things). Vata types have a greater need of calm and concentration. Pitta types need to spend more time in Nature and should favor alkaline foods.

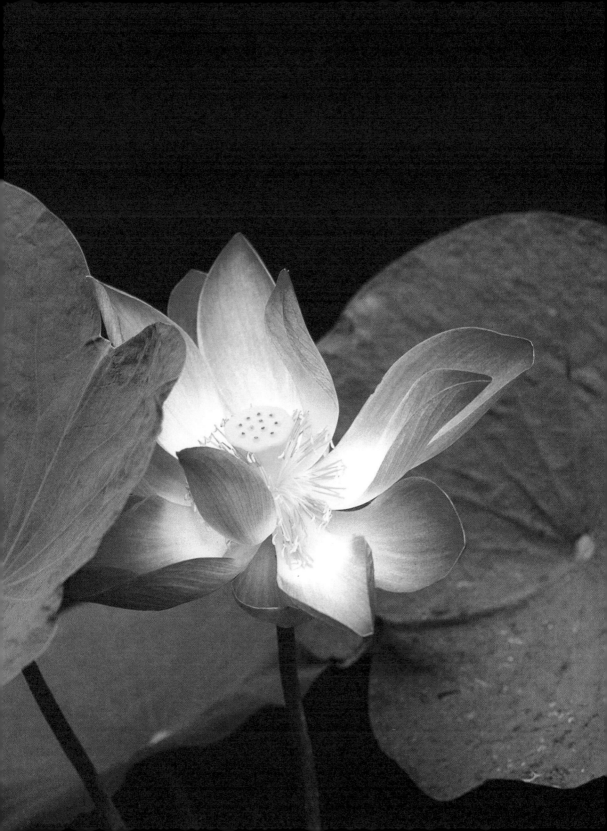

AYURVEDA IN
A SPA SETTING

By the time we returned to Paris, Nathalie and I were well versed in a wide variety of traditional therapies from the world's most culturally rich countries. So we decided to open a spa that would combine all of these therapies – an ideal wellness and beauty center situated in the very heart of the Paris Opera district. The big question now was how to adapt these therapies, massage techniques and beauty rituals for use in a spa environment.

In all of the different cultures that we visited, massage was practiced in the home or village setting, in temples with monks officiating and in so-called Ayurveda clinics under the supervision of physicians as part of an overall treatment plan.

Then there were the cosmetics products, all of them inspired by traditional beauty secrets based on natural ingredients and age-old folk remedies (plants, resins, vegetable oils, minerals, etc.). Virgin sesame oil, for instance, is a mainstay of Ayurveda – but we wouldn't have dreamed of using it in our bathroom, never mind a Parisian spa. Picture a wet dachshund and it gives you some idea of how oily and sticky sesame oil makes your hair looks.

So we enlisted the expert help of Dr Ghanashyam Marda and Dr Francine Vaution, a pharmaceutical consultant specializing in formulation, and set to work isolating the individual fatty acids from these oils, looking to produce "cocktails" of refined Ayurvedic oils that were easily absorbed and left no greasy after-feel. Marrying old and new was quite a feat – crossing traditional knowledge with state-of-the-art cosmetics technology to create products that matched customer expectations. Safe, effective products that made for a sensual spa experience tailored to the specific tastes of the Western city dweller.

Likewise with the massages themselves we found a way of retaining all the complexity of the ancient techniques without, as in India, letting therapists clad in heavy-duty waxed aprons drown their client in four liters of oil …

Oils and massage for the body, mind and skin

Ayurveda uses oils as the massage medium between the body undergoing the massage and the spa-therapist's hands. Oils facilitate techniques such as kneading, lymphatic drainage, vibration and quick tapping movements on the skin and joints. Our oils contain vitamins and essential fatty acids (Omega 3, 6, 9). Their components help the heat to penetrate without evaporating, allowing the effects of the massage to permeate throughout the body.

In India, they use oils every day to stay healthy – on the body, on the hair and particularly on the nose and in the nostrils to prevent dryness. Oils are used to clean the ears and eyes (strengthen the eyes too) and rubbed into the navel to ward off dryness and improve a weak digestion. Massaging and caring for the navel is particularly recommended in Ayurveda since the umbilicus lies at the center of a 72,000-strong network of subtle nerves (nadis) that connect with the rest of the body.

OIL

Olea *is the Latin word for oil,*
as in Olea Europaea
meaning olive tree and also
oleaginous or oily.

It is always best to start with cold pressed organic vegetable oils.

Our "Cinq Mondes Huile Universelle Ayurvédique" combines the unique properties of three oils: sesame, neem and frankincense.

MASSAGE OILS

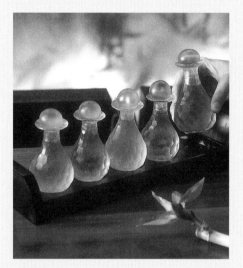

Sesame seed oil

This is the medicinal oil most widely used in India for therapeutic massage. In Hindu mythology, sesame seed is symbolic of immortality, which says a lot about the beneficial effects of sesame seed oil on the skin and bodily health. Sesame oil is unctuous, heavy, bitter and astringent and contains two valuable natural anti-oxidants: sesamol and sesamolin. It also contains minerals such as iron, phosphorous, magnesium, copper, salicylic acid and calcium. Its linoleic acid and lecithin content has a beneficial effect on the endocrine glands, neurons (nerve cells) and brain cells. High in amino acids, sesame oil is also important for brain function.

Neem oil

Neem oil is famous in India for its almost magical effects. The neem or Indian lilac is usually found growing in every village, considered a sacred tree and so revered for its wondrous properties that rural Indians call it the "healing tree" or "village pharmacy." Neem oil is a popular home remedy for minor cuts and scrapes as it accelerates wound healing to a quite astonishing degree. Rich in essential fatty acids, amino acids and vitamin E, neem oil is used in skin care oils for its dermatological, anti-inflammatory and hydrating properties, helping to sooth and soften the skin.

Frankincense (Boswellia) oil

Unusually for an essential oil, frankincense oil is not extracted from seeds or plants. It is in fact distilled from the resin of trees of the genus Boswellia, used in incense and pharmaceutical products. The raw resin, also known as Olibanum, is burnt to nourish the spirit and achieve higher consciousness in meditation. So you can see that massaging the body with a frankincense oil-based medium will produce an effect on the mind and body alike. Ayurvedic medicine has always set great store by frankincense oil in the treatment of rheumatic disorders and inflammation of the gastrointestinal and respiratory tracts. Frankincense oil was recently rediscovered by Western scientists and shown to possess powerful healing properties with no known side effects. Quite apart from its benefits for the skin and muscles, frankincense oil also has a very particular soothing smell that makes it ideal for use in massage oil.

SEASONAL MASSAGE OIL RECIPES

In every traditional culture, oil is considered a sacred product whatever the plant of origin. Oil is used in food preparation, massage, medicinal remedies, household cleaning products and also perfumery. Oil is extracted from fruit (olives, corn), nuts (argan nuts, hazelnuts, walnuts), and seeds (linseed, grape seeds). Every base oil has its own particular energy (calming, tonic, soothing, mentally stimulating ...). Oils are used in Ayurveda depending on energy type and the season.

Spring

(DOMINANT DOSHAS, KAPHA, MUCUS AND PITTA, BILE)

- 2 cups sesame oil;
- 2 tablespoons almond oil;
- 1 spoonful neem oil.

Summer

(DOMINANT DOSHA, PITTA, BILE)

- 2 cups coconut oil;
- 2 tablespoons wheat germ oil;
- 2 tablespoons sandalwood oil.

Fall

(DOMINANT DOSHA, VATA, WIND)

- 2 cups sesame oil;
- 2 tablespoons rose oil;
- 2 tablespoons castor oil.

Winter

(DOMINANT DOSHAS, VATA, WIND AND KAPHA, MUCUS)

- 2 cups olive oil;
- 2 tablespoons wheat germ oil;
- 2 tablespoons sweet almond oil;
- a few drops cardamom oil.

Abhyanga: massage that harmonizes the body

Every year I attend an Ayurvedic retreat at Sri Sri Ravi Shankar's ashram in Bangalore (Indian state of Karnataka). I go there to rebalance my own Vata constitution but also to further my understanding of the process itself. For some 15 years now we have been working with Dr Ghanashyam Marda to provide effective spa treatments that re-harmonize the flow of vital energy in the three body types.

Dr Marda began by teaching us Abhyanga: the best-known of Ayurvedic massage, producing the most "generalized" effects. It entails two hundred movements that rebalance the muscles and stimulate the energetic pathways – kneading, percussion and deep gliding strokes along the muscle fibers. Abhyanga improves circulation, restores the flow of energy, tones muscles and reduces tensions. It is unrivaled as a remedy for fatigue, helping to calm a restless mind and generally sooth and ground the body.

Hence my use of the word "generalized" to describe Abhyanga. It just happens to suit all constitutional types: toning Kapha types, soothing tense Pitta types and harmonizing body and mind to calm the restless mind that comes from a Vata imbalance. You could say that Abhyanga has something for everybody, which is why we recommend it to all of our Cinq Mondes clients regardless of country or climate.

The medium used by our spa therapists worldwide is an oil we named "Huile Universelle Ayurvédique". Suitable for all skin and body types, it combines the health benefits of sesame, frankincense and neem essential oils, rich in Omega 3, 6 and 9 fatty acids, with the soothing and rejuvenating aromas of vanilla and cardamom essential oils.

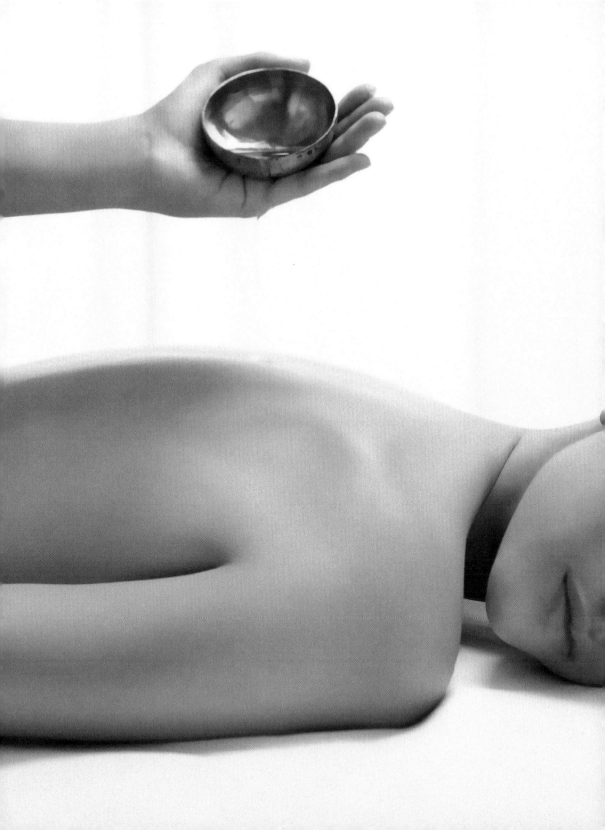

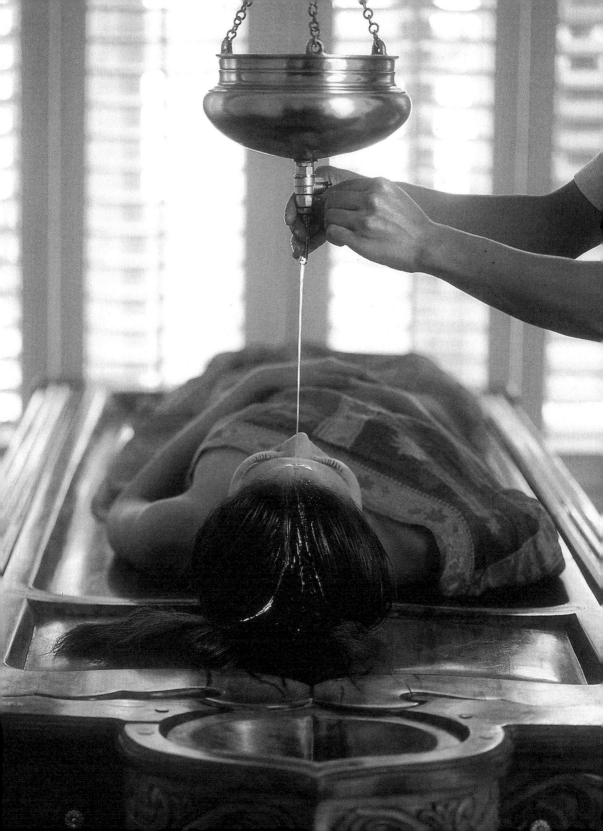

Shirodhara: massage that calms the mind

Our second Ayurvedic massage treatment is Shirodhara (from Sanskrit *dhara*, flow, and *shiro*, head). Also known as The Royal Treatment, Shirodhara was originally reserved for the nobility, maharajahs and maharanis. It involves trickling warm sesame oil in between the temples, passing over the center of the brow or "third eye" as it is known in Hinduism. The oil is poured from a very elegant copper vessel, which is suspended from a stand for ease of use and greater precision. The therapist's skill lies in swinging this vessel back and forth across the brow so that the oil flows in a steady, continuous stream from the (standard size) hole at the bottom of the vessel – which is a lot harder than it looks.

This continuous flow of warm oil over the forehead induces a state of absolute relaxation, not to say downright sleepiness, which is obviously hugely therapeutic for excitable Pitta and Vata types. Shirodhara is king when it comes to quieting the mind and tuning out distractions. It brings an inner peace that is the perfect antidote to the hustle and bustle of modern life

We offer this highly specialized form of treatment in the 15 largest Cinq Mondes spas in ten countries: in France at our Paris, Lyon, Nantes and Marseilles spas; in Switzerland at the Beau Rivage Palace, Lausanne; in Monaco at the Monte Carlo Bay; in Belgium at the Hôtel Dolce La Hulpe, Brussels; in Dubai at the Kempinski Hotel and Residences, Palm Jumeirah; in the USA at our spas in Carmel (California) and Long Beach; in Morocco at the Club Med resort in Marrakech; in Mauritius at La Plantation d'Albion and the Sugar Beach Hotel; and in Qatar at the Wyndham Grand Regency Doha.

Shirodhara requires on-going training by our therapists as it ends with a gentle scalp and head massage that requires very precise hand movements.

Udarabhyanga: an ancient method of detoxification

Ayurvedic medicine attaches great importance to the stomach or belly (Sanskrit, *udar*), seeing it as the body's central cog, the vital energy center. Often called the second brain, the stomach is directly connected to the first brain – the two "talk" to each other. There are more than one hundred million neurons embedded in the walls of our gut. If our stomach hurts, so do our body and our spirit. The hormones secreted by the stomach control the digestive and elimination system. But the stomach also houses an important microbial system composed of some 200 billion bacteria and fungi that are vital to life. Last but by no means least, the stomach is the center of emotion –the expression "to have a knot in your stomach" says it all.

Udarabhyanga, or abdomen/belly massage, takes its inspiration from Panchakarma: a five-fold Ayurveda cleansing therapy that places great emphasis on caring for the stomach. Udarabhyanga consists of deep, gliding strokes to relax the tissues; lymph drainage and vibration techniques to promote the elimination of toxins; and strokes that generate heat to stimulate blood flow. When used in conjunction with a balanced diet for your dosha body type, Udarabhyanga works wonders, detoxifying the body and making you feel lighter in body and mind ...

Udvartana treatment for slimming and detox

The quest for slimness, setting aside aesthetic considerations, forms part of the holistic vision of Ayurveda, seen as the shedding of unnecessary ballast through purification and detoxification.

At Cinq Mondes, we have revived a traditional recipe based on gram flour, which is known for its cleansing properties. When used as an exfoliant, our product leaves the skin exceptionally soft. Repeated applications rid the skin of all underlying impurities, smoothing out any rough areas, removing blemishes and letting the skin "breathe." The Udvartana treatment itself comprises highly effective synergistic techniques that commence with a series of deep breaths to bring awareness of the body as a whole. This is followed by a warm wrap based on ginger and Indian gooseberry (*Embellica officinalis*) that stimulates microcirculation, eliminates toxins and helps to remodel the body and figure. The final stage consists of a toning massage to stimulate the circulation, then lymphatic drainage to promote elimination and restore the energies.

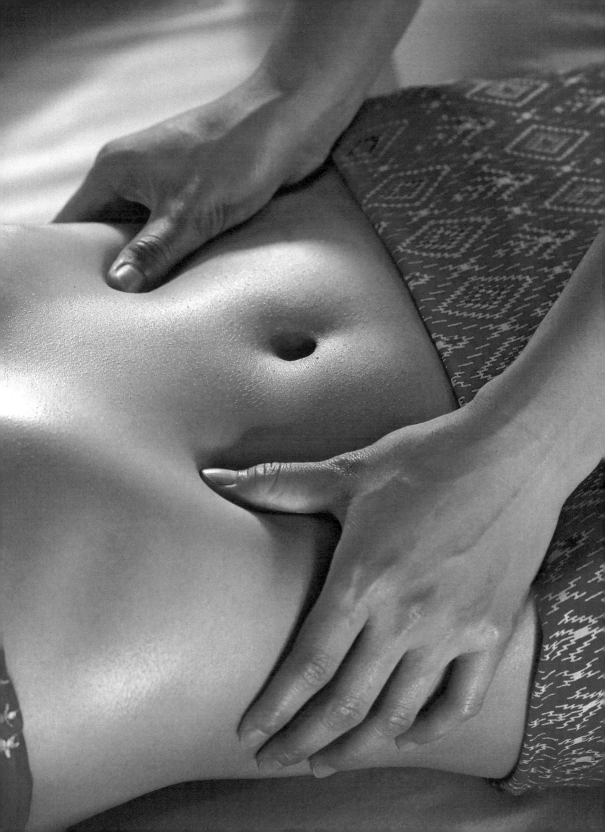

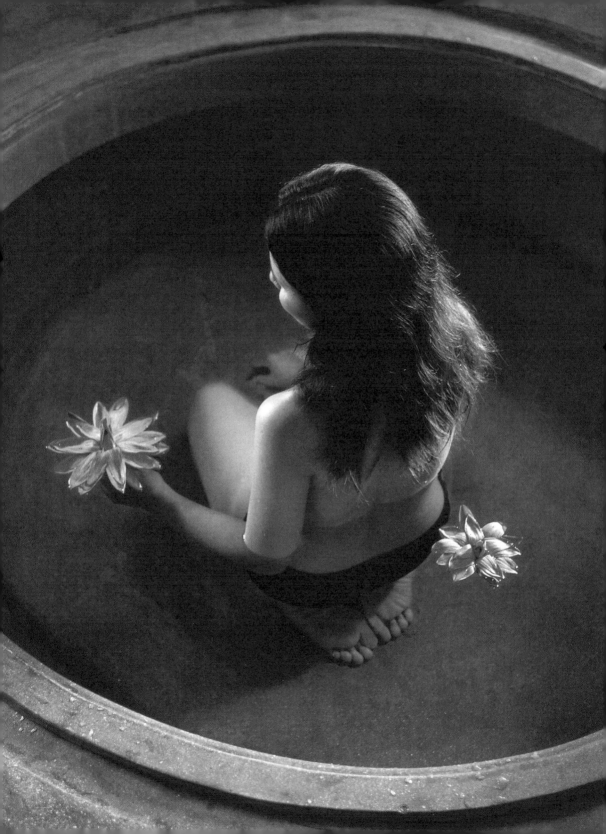

AYURVEDIC CLINICS AT THE CINQ MONDES "HEALTH AND WELLNESS RETREATS"

In the course of my wellness research, it occurred to me that what was missing from our Western lifestyles was the kind of retreat you find in India, complete with massage, meditation, yoga, nutritional advice and so forth. So I decided to make this a part of the Cinq Mondes mission – invent something halfway between tradition and the latest spa technology.

Ayurveda offered me a wide range of possibilities, particularly considering that all of the treatments administered during a seven-day retreat are aimed at restoring wholeness. They rebalance energy flows, eliminate toxins and purify the body and mind through deep relaxation techniques whose effects extend all the way to the cellular texture of the skin. In short, they make you "feel comfortable in your own skin."

Our whole approach at Cinq Mondes is founded on precisely this quest for holistic wellness. With that in mind, three of our spas have actually evolved beyond traditional beauty and cosmetics centers into full-on "Health and Wellness Retreats:" at the Beau Rivage Hotel, Lausanne; the Kempinski Hotel, Dubai; and the Long Beach Hotel, Mauritius, surrounded by tropical rain forest. All three offer a balanced health and wellness program encompassing five areas and five dimensions:

• **Spa treatments plus "Ayurvedic health weeks:"** seven days of (doubly therapeutic) beauty and wellness rituals that care for the body, the skin and the spirit;

• **Dietary guidelines** but also an invitation to the "slow life". There is nothing wrong with liking your food! Eating provides energy for the body but also the spirit. In our accelerating world, we have forgotten the golden rules of good eating – how to eat to increase vitality while also achieving a wonderful sense of lightness. Take for example the rule that eating slowly, chewing every mouthful thoroughly, is the first step to proper digestion. There was a time when an egg timer would be placed on the table as an invitation to slow down ... Slow eating makes for better digestion but it also celebrates the joys of life, reacquainting us with forgotten tastes, colors and flavors. It is the high road to balancing your mind, body and spirit.

– Sleep therapy, focusing on treatments like Shirodhara (a sovereign remedy for jetlag). All of the bedrooms in our partner hotels offer a choice of pillows misted with Cinq Mondes Eau Egyptienne, which combines 11 essential oils including juniper, nutmeg, cloves and lotus flower. I discovered the formula on the walls of the temple of Edfu – the selfsame formula as was used to blend the perfume for Queen Hatshepsut 35 centuries ago, described by the Greek writer and philosopher Plutarch as "allaying anxieties and brightening dreams." A good night's sleep is a necessity, not a luxury. When the mind shuts down for the night, our brain "replays" the events of the day and stores the highlights. It also produces growth hormones that play a vital role in cell regeneration or, at the risk of repeating myself, in making us "comfortable in our own skin."

– Physical activity and yoga: the art of yoga (Sanskrit for "union" or "method of discipline") brings mind and body together. It is an integral part of Ayurvedic medicine, now practiced by people around the world including some 37 million Americans. Yoga exercises the body, calms the mind and teaches us to control prana, the life force. It encompasses hundreds of poses and breathing techniques that are adapted for students of different levels, bringing benefits that are apparent from the very first sessions.

– Hydrotherapy: water is the energy of life. It is the medium that surrounds our first nine months and the element to which we are instinctively drawn thereafter to cleanse the mind and body. So it is well worth taking the time to luxuriate in water and become fully aware of its healing energies. Our hydrotherapy facilities are designed to tone and relax at the same time, alternating massage jets, cold experience rooms (ice fountain) and hot tubs (Turkish baths set to around 110 degrees Fahrenheit).

Every day at Cinq Mondes we observe first hand how working on the subtle balance between the soma and the psyche serves to rejuvenate and restore the "whole person," make them feel "comfortable in their own skin" right down to the cellular level. We know from experience that mind–body balance combined with regular application of the patented vegetable oils and ingredients contained in Cinq Mondes cosmetics make it possible to prolong the youth of the body, the mind and the skin.

 Restoring balance, bringing body, spirit and breathing back into harmony, is the vital link between the soma and the psyche. "

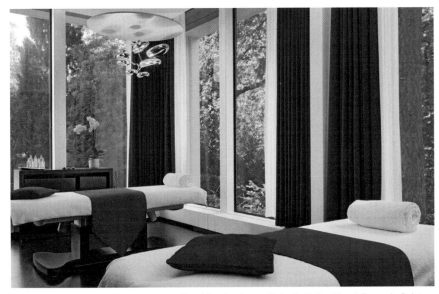

Cinq Mondes Spa at Dolce la Hulpe Hotel, Brussels, Belgium

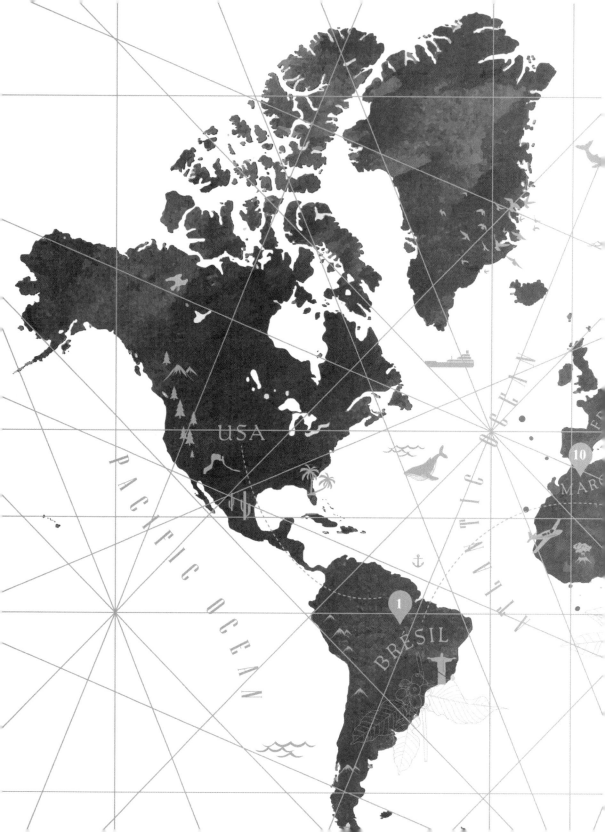

3

HEALTH AND
HOLISTIC BEAUTY:
THE TEACHINGS OF
SRI SRI RAVI SHANKAR

___

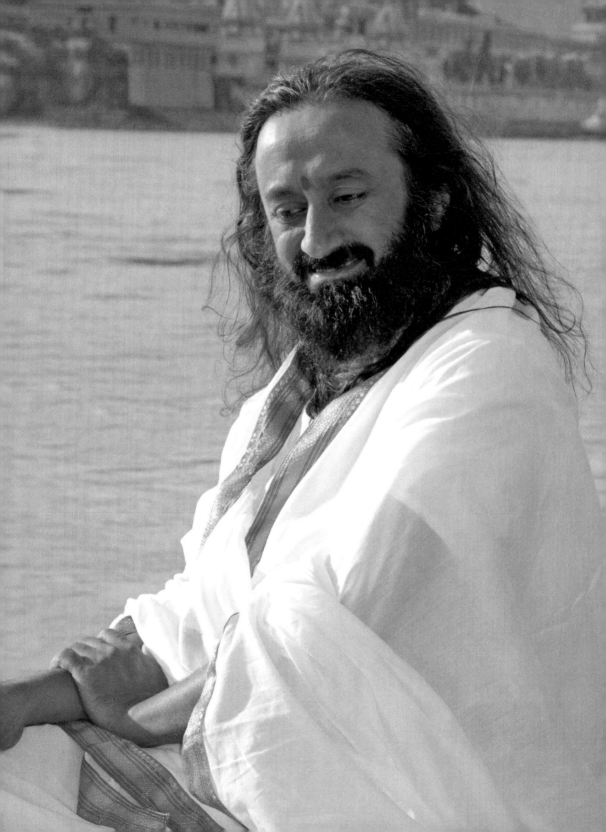

"Breathing is not so much important as inevitable! To understand the intimate link between the breath, the body and the spirit: simply stop breathing!"

SRI SRI RAVI SHANKAR

After mixing with the Indian community in Bayswater for so many years, I always sensed that breathing was one of the keys to wellbeing and concentration, the invisible thread linking body and mind. In 2000, I had the pleasure to discover the teachings of Sri Sri Ravi Shankar, an Indian spiritual leader who combines uncommon erudition with a wonderfully straightforward approach to teaching that revolves around energizing breathing exercises called Sudarshan Kriya (kriya: purifying action, sudarshan: clear vision).

According to the teachings of Sri Sri Ravi Shankar, every emotion imprints a particular rhythm on our breathing. So by mastering our breathing, we can take back control of our emotions – cast off negative feelings and boost our level of energy (prana). Medical research into these exercises has shown that they yield considerable benefits for our physical and mental wellbeing. They reduce stress by lowering levels of the stress hormone, cortisol; boost our immune system; relieve anxiety and depression; and improve our ability to concentrate.

Since 1982 Sri Sri Ravi Shankar's NGO, Art of Living, has taught these powerful and liberating breathing techniques to more than 20 million people. Art of Living is also active on humanitarian fronts, promoting such causes as education for underprivileged children, good prison practice and decent housing, and also supporting people who suffer from post-traumatic stress following natural disasters. I find this kind of breathing a great help. It allows me to be dynamic in my work but also to let go mentally and spiritually – it was invaluable when I was setting up Cinq Mondes.

SRI SRI RAVI SHANKAR,
YOGA TEACHER
AND SPIRITUAL LEADER

I first met Sri Sri Ravi Shankar at one of his ashrams in Canada, not long after leaving on our voyage of discovery, then again at the end of our tour a year later, at his Bangalore ashram in India. Revered as a sage, Sri Sri Ravi Shankar is a Nobel Peace Prize nominee and the brains behind the Art of Living Foundation, a volunteer-based non-governmental organization established in 1982. Since then, it has spread to more than 150 countries and currently mobilizes some two million volunteers. The Foundation plays a key role in the promotion of yoga teaching, meditation, healthcare, decent housing and education for underprivileged children (a program supported by Cinq Mondes that provides annual funding for primary schools). The Art of Living Foundation also supports the victims of natural disasters (such as Hurricane Katrina and the Gujarat earthquake) by providing techniques for overcoming post-traumatic stress disorder. On a personal level, Sri Sri Ravi Shankar is a regular speaker at UNESCO and Davos, and recently played a role in brokering a peace deal between the Columbian government and FARC.

I knew none of this when I actually met the great man himself. But from the very beginning I was struck by his extraordinarily calming presence – by the quality of the silence that reigned when he was teaching yoga and how relaxed one felt after his guided meditations. Then there was his minute attention to detail, which might be a particular flower arrangement or the way you were feeling that day.

I remember, for instance, the time when 15 of us were attending a brief question-and-answer session with Sri Sri following a group meditation. I was supposed to come third but in all the excitement I couldn't think of a single question to ask – so he simply "skipped my turn" and addressed himself to the next person.

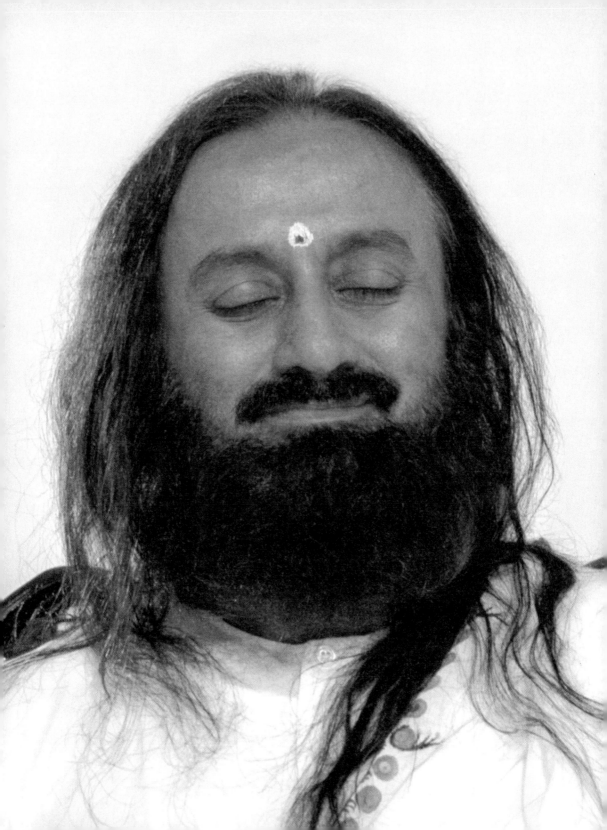

I realized later, as I listened to the other questions and answers, that what I should have asked was this: "What's the best way to get rid of unwanted thoughts while practicing?" But by then the session was coming to an end and there was nothing I could do except feel sorry for myself. Or so I thought, because it was just then that Sri Sri turned to me and asked with a mischievous smile: "What about you? Didn't you want to ask me something?" I was speechless – well not quite. I did at least manage to blurt out my burning question. "Are these thoughts useful?" he asked. No, I replied. "So just drop them," he said.

" *– Are these thoughts useful?*

– No.

– So just drop them. **"**

It was his first invitation to the art of letting go – a concept that underpins his teachings and that has helped me to grow ever since.

For some 35 years now, Sri Sri Ravi Shankar has been teaching mind-body breathing and meditation techniques whose effects extend all the way to the cellular texture of the skin. But before we look at these in more detail, let us first take a closer look at this Indian wise man himself. In 2016, to celebrate the thirty-fifth anniversary of his NGO, he organized a "World Culture Festival" in Delhi that drew three and a half million people from 84 countries plus 37,000 musicians and dancers who performed on an immense stage measuring 21,000m2 (around 26,000 square yards). It was rightly hailed as an immense effort to promote world peace.

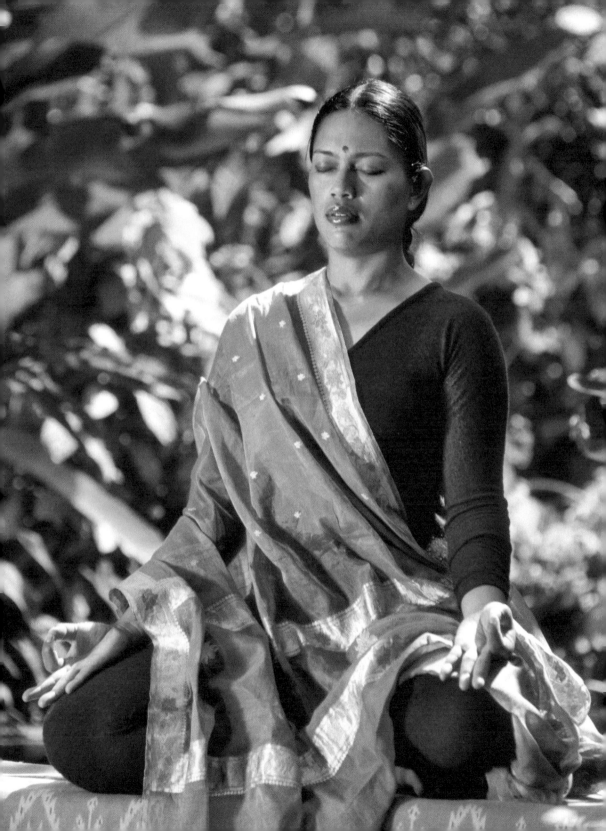

An intellectual and spiritual journey

Sri Sri Ravi Shankar was born in southern India in 1956, to an affluent Brahman family that donated most of its wealth to good works and most of its time to the pursuit of art and spiritual growth. By the age of four, Sri Sri was able to recite parts of the Ashtavakra Gita and the Bhagavad Gita, ancient Sanskrit scriptures, by heart. His mother would often find him deep in meditation while his friends were playing football outside the family house. He was taught the Vedic texts by Gandhi's Sanskrit teacher, Dr Sudhakar Chaturvedi, who though he gave up teaching after the Mahatma's death changed his mind after meeting the then four-year old Ravi Shankar.

By the age of 17, Ravi Shankar had not just completed the traditional syllabus but also obtained a doctorate in physical science. In the words of His Holiness the Dalai Lama: "By successfully reconciling his scientific education with his Vedic instruction, Sri Sri Ravi Shankar has found a pathway to knowledge that meets contemporary needs." In 1982, following a ten-day period of fasting and silence, he devised the Sudarshan Kriya, a powerful breathing meditation technique, and drew together the principles that would shape his teaching.

A universal art of living

The Art of Living Foundation (www.artofliving.org) was established that same year to provide tools to relieve individual stress and ultimately achieve world peace. Since then Sri Sri Ravi Shankar has spent his life traveling the globe, visiting more than 150 cities every year to give talks at international venues (the United Nations, the European Parliament and Davos among others) and meet the world's top political and religious leaders.

Though he is now a globally revered spiritual leader he still somehow manages to remain close to his followers. Whenever he sees me, this man who meets hundreds of thousands of people every year always asks me for news about "your Cinq Mondes spas." But a prodigious memory is by no means the only quality of this master teacher. His disciples call him "Guruji", from the Sanskrit word "guru" for "master" or "teacher". The name may seem a bit intimidating to we Westerners, not to say cliquey, but as Sri Sri explains: "No-one would think of learning to play the guitar or the piano without a teacher or guru. It's the same when it comes to mastering stress or the subtle art of balancing your mind and body. A teacher is as least as important here as when learning music."

In 1986, Sri Sri Ravi Shankar's prowess as a teacher won him the title of *Yoga Shiromani* ("supreme jewel of yoga"), an honor bestowed on him by the then President of India. His vast body of teachings is shaped by three main factors: age-old knowledge of the intimate workings of the human mind; a form of yoga accessible to the typical Westerner; and above all, unique breathing techniques that eliminate stress, mental agitation and anxiety while also bringing equanimity, serenity and remarkable mental clarity. All of this also helps to reduce oxidative stress, which is one of the main causes of premature skin aging.

Unique breathing techniques

Beyond words, it is the role of the master to provide tools and techniques for progress. It should be clear by now that for Sri Sri Ravi Shankar, breathing is the driving force behind personal transformation. He is the architect of a particular breathing technique called Sudarshan Kriya, which means "proper vision by purifying action." Sudarshan Kriya works through poses and breathing rhythms with powerful effects, helping to release negative emotions and restore the subtle balance between body and mind. As a practitioner myself, I can vouch for its efficiency. Sri Sri Ravi Shankar, apart from teaching the mechanics of the technique, is also best placed to explain its spiritual benefits.

INNER BALANCE OUTER BEAUTY

SRI SRI RAVI SHANKAR

In what way do the effects of breathing influence the skin at the cellular level?

Breathing removes most of the toxins from the body. Breathing is the link between body and mind. Breathing techniques such as Sudarshan Kriya exert an influence on the mind-body complex. Many studies have been devoted to understanding that impact. Beyond its effects on the endocrine system, Sudarshan Kriya has been shown to produce changes right down at the genetic level. In one particular study, it was shown to have a positive impact on gene expression, changing more than 300 genes in the human body.

What is the link between Inner Peace and Outer Beauty?

Feelings of inner peace and happiness are reflected in the way a person looks, acts and behaves in general. The reason we all find children so beautiful is because they are so pure and innocent on the inside. Our mind is a sea of thoughts and feelings, some good, some bad, which come and go all the time. Over-identification with those thoughts and feelings makes us feel blocked, inadequate. But if we look deeper inside ourselves we find only calm space within. That space that appears inside us is our own vast consciousness, which is the embodiment of bliss and love. Then we see that the quality of the consciousness has expanded beyond its limitations, and therein lies our true nature. Therein lies Beauty. For external beauty, we put on things; for real beauty we have to discard those things. For external beauty we have to have make-up; for real beauty we have only to realize that we are already made-up.

Here again we see the mark of our mischievous guru – in this amusing but meaningful play on words, "make-up" and "made-up", signifying quite different things depending on the context.

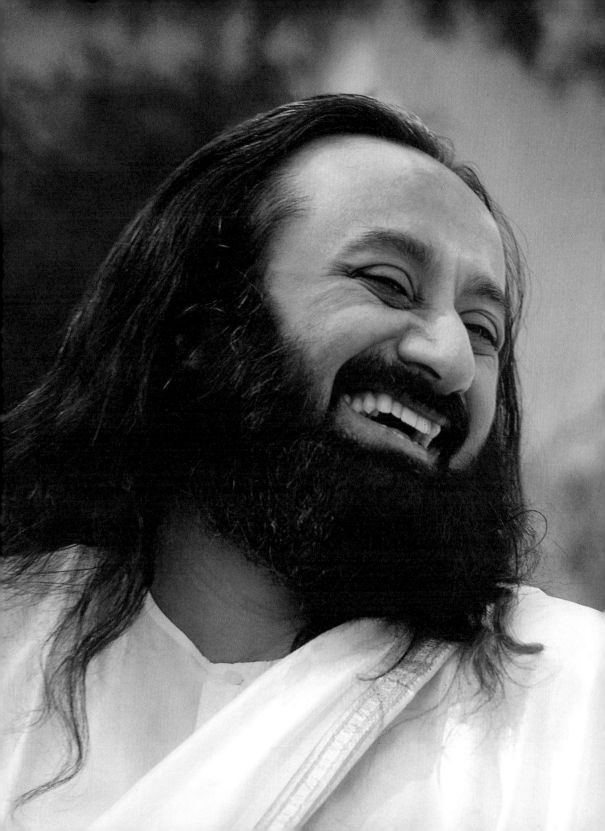

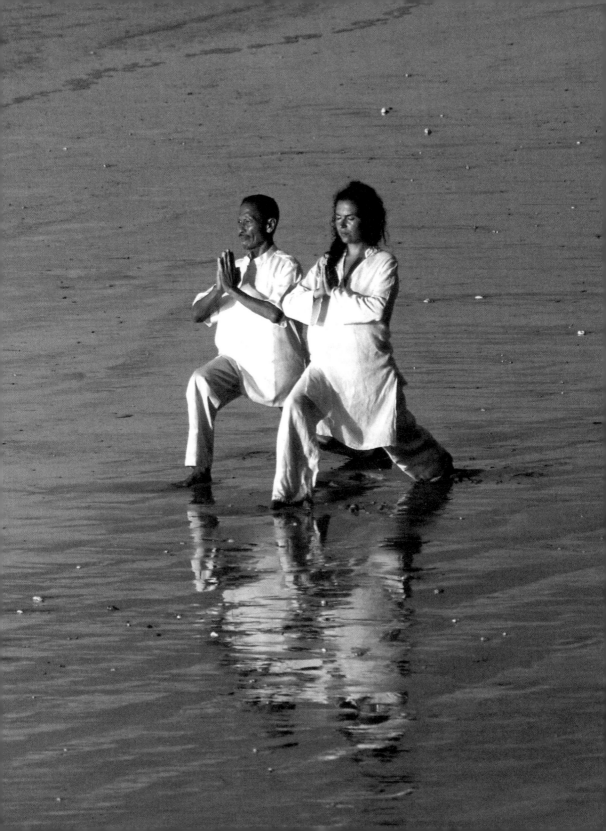

BREATHING,
THE BODY-MIND
LINK

Sri Sri makes use of another wonderful comparison to describe the interaction between the body and mind: "If the mind is a kite, the breath is the string. The longer the string, the higher the kite can fly. Just as you control a kite with the string, so by working the breath you can start to have some control over your mind."

> " *Breathing bridges the gap between feelings and the body. Changing the rhythm of the breath calms the mind and liberates it from negative thinking.* "

SRI SRI RAVI SHANKAR

His breathing techniques were invaluable at the beginning, when we were building our Paris Opera spa. I used them to overcome the negative feelings that overwhelmed me whenever we hit a new problem – which happened about ten times a day. For instance, we hadn't bargained on having to drill through a six-foot thick wall – nor expected the Turkish bath to flood when the water was turned on.

Working on the breath grounds you in the "here and now," in what matters. And a return to essentials has never been more important than today, in a society suffering from information overload and social media addiction. Most of our experiences are purely imaginary, virtual not real, cutting us off from our emotions – emotions that must be felt to the full to be truly liberating. Breathing is particularly helpful in this regard.

So too is yoga, a Vedic discipline that aims to reunify the physical, psychological and spiritual dimensions of our being through physical exercise. Attention to the breath plays a particularly central role in yoga practice. The writings (*sutras*) of Patanjali, one of the great masters and theoreticians of yoga, refer to eight limbs or branches of yoga – eight stages on the road to happiness and inner peace. The fourth limb is Pranayama or the art of breathing, a combination of two Sanskrit words: *yama* meaning restraint or control, and *prana*, the vital energy or life force.

Breathing helps to relieve emotional and mental stress and reduce levels of the stress hormone, cortisol, thereby counteracting the oxidative stress that accelerates cellular aging.

YOGA

The word "yoga" is rooted in the ancient Sanskrit word "jug", meaning bind, join, unite, bring together, with particular reference to uniting the body, mind and soul. Practicing yoga restores our integrity as human beings by putting us in touch with our inner selves.

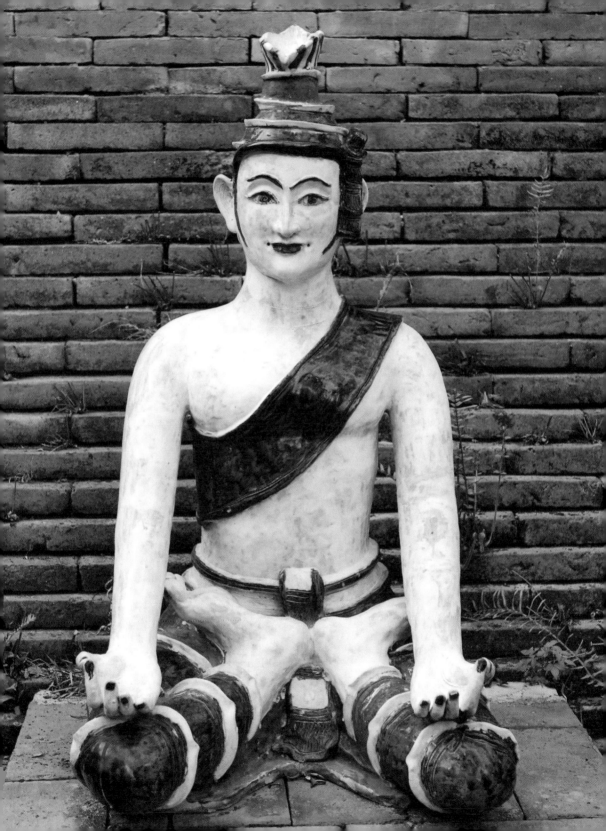

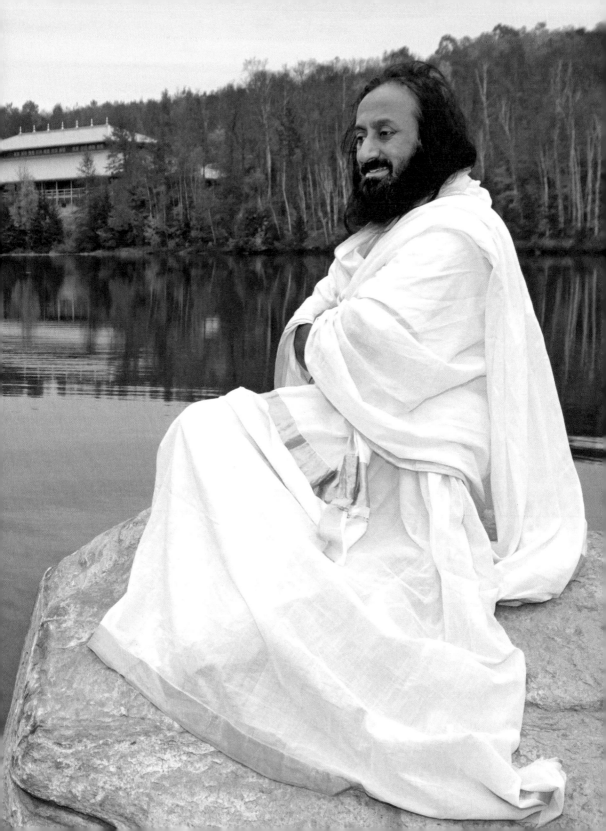

" *The breath is the connecting link between the inner world of silence and the outer world of activity. Working on the breath helps us to control the mind because breath is more tangible than mind.* "

SRI SRI RAVI SHANKAR

From controlling your thoughts to cell nirvana

There can be few things more difficult than trying to control your thoughts ... with those self-same thoughts. Our mind runs rampant with thoughts, and it is an illusion to believe you can think yourself into another way of thinking – whatever the claims made by fashionable American practitioners of cognitive behavioral therapy. People who try and force themselves to think in a certain way are like cats chasing their own tails ...

The breath offers us an alternative approach – indirect but far more effective. The breath is the invisible thread between body and mind. Because breathing oxygenates every cell in our body, it restores the body's tissue repair system and maintains homeostasis – that perfect state of equilibrium within a cell that I call its "nirvana." Homeostasis is the key to staying young: young body, young mind, and yes, even young skin. It gives a whole new meaning to the expression "feeling comfortable in your own skin."

YOGA
BREATHING EXERCISES

The following three poses play with this principle of breath as the life force. I find them deeply relaxing and do not for one moment doubt their rejuvenating effects – all the more reason to share them with you now.

I. THE JOY OF BREATHING

Stand with your feet shoulder-width apart, arms by your side. Inhale deeply and vigorously through your nose and raise your arms above your head in a "V" shape, stretching the respiratory muscles and opening up the solar plexus. Bring the arms behind the ears as you finish inhaling and tilt your head very slightly backward.

As you exhale, bring the arms forward and cross them over the chest, chin tucked in.

Repeat some ten times, paying attention to the sensations aroused by the air as it travels to the lungs – through the nose and throat, around the collarbones and the solar plexus, all the way to the navel.

Practicing this exercise regularly offers many benefits. It increases lung capacity, stretches and improves the flexibility of the thoracic and abdominal muscles, and relaxes the solar plexus (seat of the emotions). The more you practice, the greater the benefits, including stimulating the connection between the respiratory system and the brain, and between the brain and the stomach or "second brain".

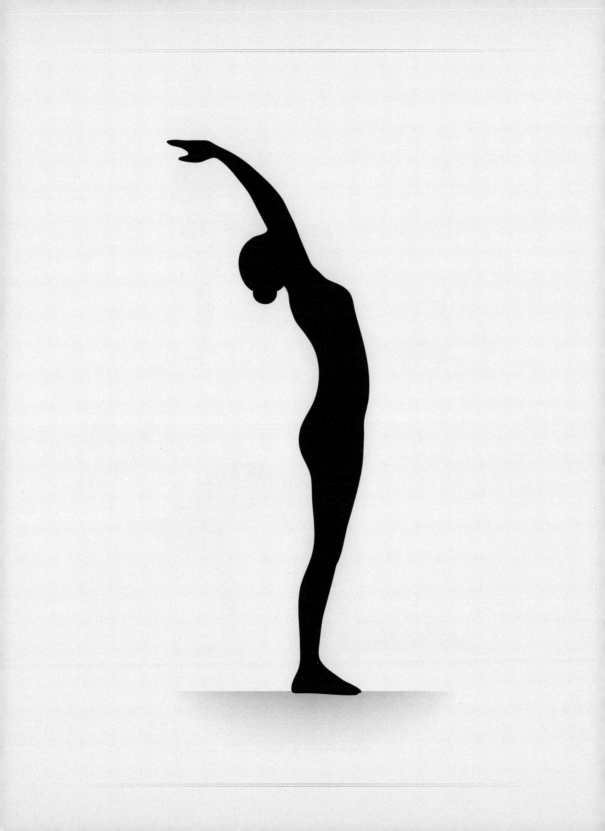

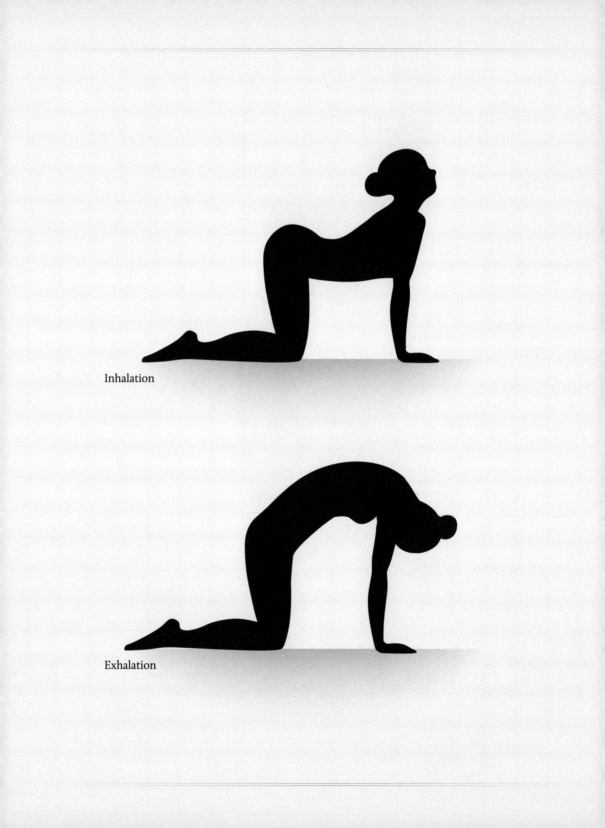

Inhalation

Exhalation

2. BREATHING IN CAT POSE

Cat pose (like cobra and monkey pose, to mention but two) is one of the many asanas that were inspired by observation of the natural/animal world. It works on the respiratory system (rib cage, diaphragm, etc) while also improving spinal flexibility. Cat pose is practiced in two stages, hollowing the back on the inhalation, and rounding the back on the exhalation.

• Stage One: Inhalation.
Position yourself on all fours, hands directly under your shoulders, knees set directly below your hips. As you inhale, arch your back so the belly drops toward the floor and push into the floor with your arms to lift the head, tilting the chin upward. With the lungs filled to capacity, hold the breath for a few seconds.

• Stage Two: Exhalation.
As you exhale, tuck the pelvis underneath you to round the back like a cat, bring the chin toward the chest and suck the belly into the spine. With the lungs empty, hold the breath for a few seconds.

Repeat about ten times, paying particular attention as you inhale to the sensations aroused by the air on its way from the throat to the navel. As you exhale, be sure to empty the lungs completely by rounding the back as much as possible and tucking the chin well in.

This is another marvelous exercise. It improves spinal and pelvic flexibility, massages the internal organs and has a deeply relaxing effect on the diaphragm. It also of course improves the interaction between breathing and brain oxygenation, thereby inducing a state of deep relaxation that in turn leads to body-mind harmony and lower stress levels.

3. CHILD POSE

This important yoga pose is the perfect complement to the breathing in cat pose. Practiced directly afterwards, it induces a deep state of relaxation.

After stretching in cat, place the buttocks on the heels and lean forward, laying your torso on the thighs and extending your arms in front of you, allowing the head to rest lightly on the floor between the two arms.

Now inhale and reach the arms as far forward as you can. Then hold the breath for a few seconds before exhaling softly.

Next, sweep your arms back alongside the body, resting the hands on the ankles and relaxing the head, shoulders and neck. Remain in the pose for about 30 seconds, breathing normally, then extend the arms forward again to repeat Part One of the exercise.

Pay attention to the sensations aroused, particularly as you stretch the spine in Part One to relax the lower back. Child pose mirrors the fetal position, instilling feelings of ultimate comfort and security.

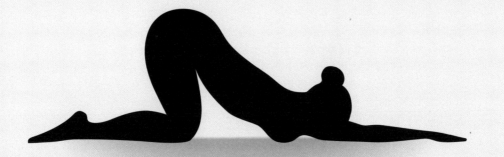

All three of these poses help to expand the ribcage for inhalation, to lengthen and stretch the spine, and to relieve pressure on the lumbar vertebra, the while giving your internal organs a wonderful massage!

The benefits of Sudarshan Kriya

Sudarshan Kriya is without a doubt the discovery that has had the greatest influence on my life, making me who I am today.

It is a very special breathing technique and an ideal prelude to meditation. I was first taught Sudarshan Kriya in 1999, just before I established Cinq Mondes, by one of the teachers at the Art of Living Foundation. The process itself is described in detail in Serge Michenaud's book on breathing, *La Pratique de la Respiration*. A shorter, 30-minute version of Sudarshan Kriya for daily use (also known as "Short Kriya") is quite sufficient to dispel negative feelings and emotions, oxygenate the entire body and "reset" the activity of the brain so that you focus on the here and now (and not on the chatter inside your head). The technique sharpens the intuition, boosts creative thinking and unclutters the mind to a quite extraordinary degree. Hence its name, Sudarshan Kriya, which is a combination of three Sanskrit words, *su, darshan and kriya* – meaning proper, vision and purifying action.

The first few years of this business were incredibly demanding physically, mentally and also emotionally. Practicing Sudarshan Kriya twice a day helped me cope. Two 30-minute sessions, one first thing in the morning and one after work, put me in a state where the problems and difficulties literally rolled off me like water off a duck's back, freeing my imagination to express itself.

Pranayama and the life force

The principles of Sudarshan Kriya were described very early by Vedic science, most notably in Patanjali's yoga sutras: "interrupt the respiratory rhythm, hold the breath, then change the rhythm of the breath to modulate prana (original life force)."

Rhythmic breathing is a fundamental principle of Sudarshan Kriya. Our body and mind are ruled by rhythms – the cardiac rhythm, sleep-wake rhythm and the rhythm of digestion, to mention but three. They might be regular or irregular but all of these rhythms are directly influenced by the primordial rhythm of breathing. Using the breath to restore rhythm to mind and body can solve a lot of problems.

There are huge benefits to be drawn from breathing, particular as 90 per cent of the toxins in our body are excreted through the lungs during exhalation. The toxins excreted through sweat, for instance, are negligible by comparison. But quite apart from removing toxins, breathing also lowers cortisol levels (the stress hormone, linked to oxidation and premature aging) and unlocks the emotions that are imprinted in cellular memory at times of trauma. According to Ayurveda, breathing drives and directs prana (energy) along the 72,000-strong network of *nadis* through which the life force circulates. The symptoms of low prana are many and varied and include apathy, self-doubt, inhibition and indecision. With daily Sudarshan Kriya practice, your energy levels skyrocket and self-doubt fades away, leaving you confident and emotionally stable.

PRANAYAMA
IN ACTION

For maximum impact, Sudarshan Kriya is preceded by three types of breathing: clavicular (shallow), thoracic (medium) and abdominal (deep). Known as prana-yamas, these serve to harmonize the body and reinforce the flow of vital energy, with rebound effects for the mind in terms of mental strength, clarity and balanced thinking.

Ujjayi breathing to overcome blockages

Before looking at these pranayamas more closely, we must first explore a way of breathing known in Sanskrit as "ujjayi pranayama", from *ud*, bondage or blockage, and jayi, conquest or victory. Ujjayi pranayama is designed to rid the body of physical and psychological blockages – for it was ever the mission of the ancient Indian sages to liberate mankind from suffering. It is hugely comforting to know that their goal was always to make us stronger, more confident and more independent.

The following extract from Serge Michenaud's *La Pratique de la Respiration* helps to understand the principle of Ujjayi breathing. "Compared to normal breathing, when the passage of the air is silent, smooth and unrestricted, Ujjayi is practiced by partially closing the glottis and gently contracting the muscles of the larynx. This creates a soft hissing sound, which comes from the throat and is felt in the windpipe and also on the soft palate."

Personally I like to compare Ujjayi breathing to a purring or light snoring sound. As the vibration in the back of the throat travels up to the limbic system (a control center for emotions and hormones), it produces a rich, deep sound that plunges you into a state of perfect relaxation.

Ujjayi breathing is routinely taught in yoga classes, Hatha and Ashtanga alike, as a way to lengthen and regulate the breath in asana practice in order to relax into the stretches. Ujjayi calms the mind and thoughts and is an ideal prelude to sleep.

Three levels of breathing to restore wholeness

Once Ujjayi breathing is mastered, you are ready to embark on the three breathing exercises of pranayama, which as we saw earlier comprise three distinct "stages" of breathing: abdominal, thoracic and clavicular.

All three are practiced in diamond pose, Vajrasana, buttocks resting on the heels, spine straight, palms of the hands on the hips (for abdominal breathing) and under the shoulders (for thoracic breathing). For clavicular breathing, bend the elbows back and point them toward the ceiling, cocking the wrists back so that the hands rest on the shoulder blades.

Each stage consists of successive respiratory cycles, performed in the following order: inhale for four counts, hold for four counts, exhale for four counts, hold for two counts. Then repeat the stage.

At each stage, inhalation draws in new energy, breath retention concentrates the life force or prana and exhalation produces a sense of relaxation, its length determining the quality and depth of the following inhalation.

These three pranayama exercises are the ideal, indeed essential prelude to Sudarshan Kriya, which engages the entire body in alternating slow and rapid breathing exercises of variable depth that optimize our ability to think clearly. They awaken the mind, sharpen our senses and enhance our intellectual and creative faculties.

MEDITATION FOLLOWS
NATURALLY FROM THESE
THREE PRANAYAMAS

After practicing Sudarshan Kriya, most people naturally "fall" into a deep state of meditation – a deep healing meditation that allows the body to repair itself and regenerate. This link with healing has been demonstrated by neuroscientists who have studied the age-old techniques of meditation. Just a few minutes of meditation serve to repair our body, mind and spirit – the effects are felt all the way down to the cellular level of the skin.

Numerous studies have been conducted in the USA, Europe and India to measure the benefits of Sudarshan Kriya. We will confine ourselves here to mentioning the research findings of Dr Brown, a member of the Columbia College of Physicians in New York: "There is sufficient evidence to consider Sudarshan Kriya yoga as a beneficial, low-risk, low-cost adjunct to the treatment of stress and stress-related medical illnesses, anxiety and depression."

We all know that stress and stress-related hormones (cortisol) accelerate aging in general and skin aging in particular. Depression changes a person's looks quite dramatically: the skin becomes like parchment and the face looks increasingly lined and careworn.

So to keep features and skin looking young, you have to consider the person as a whole. Tools such as yoga and breathing plus techniques like Sudarshan Kriya and massage serve to stimulate endorphins, not stress hormones. By boosting our well-being, they help to maintain a subtle balance between body and mind.

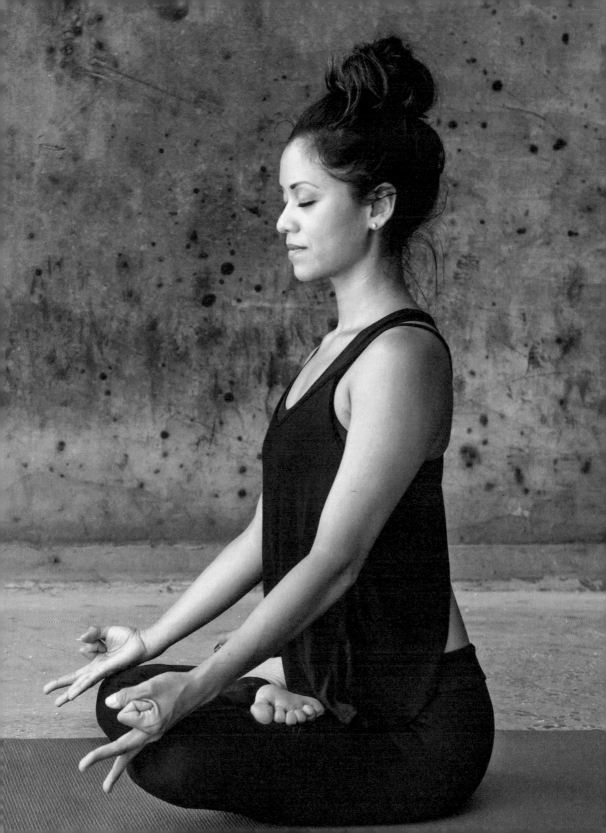

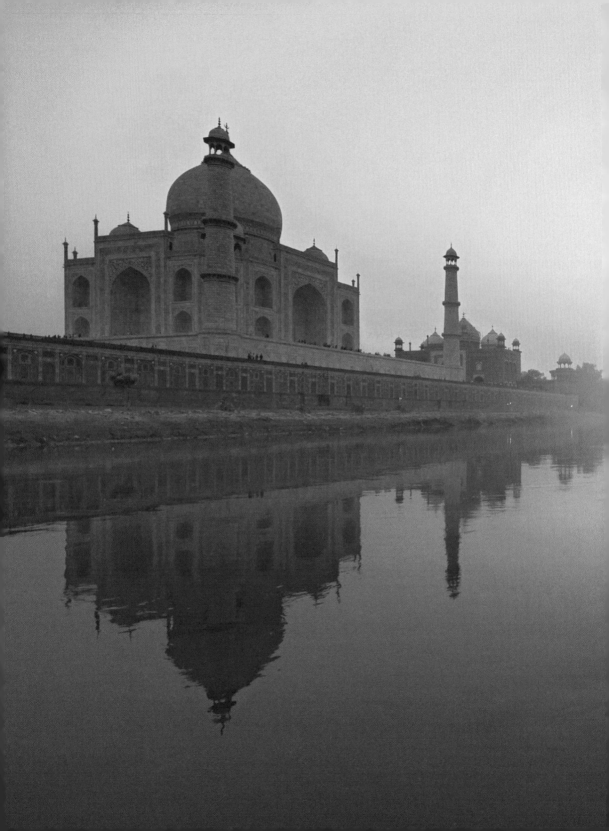

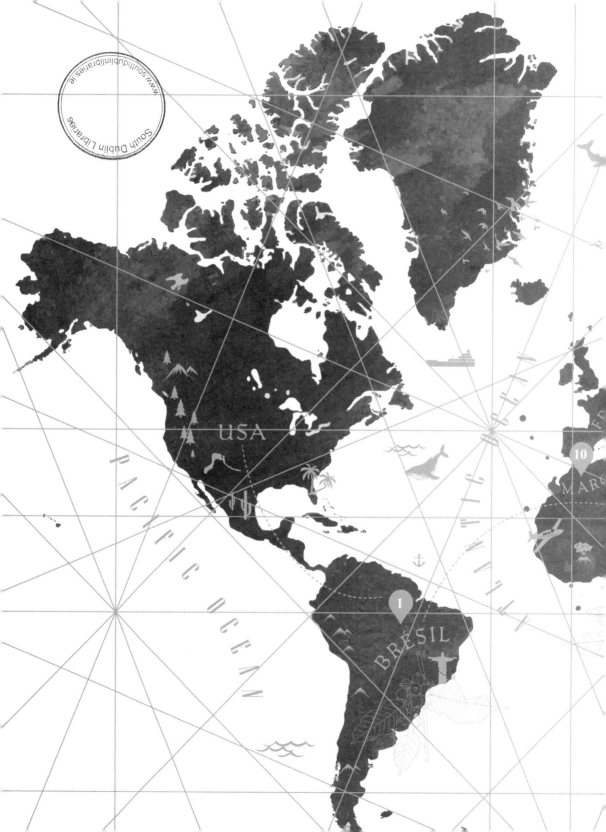

USA

PACIFIC OCEAN

ATLANTIC OCEAN

10

MAR

BRÉSIL

1

4

TOWARDS
A SKIN
DIETETICS
PROGRAM

___

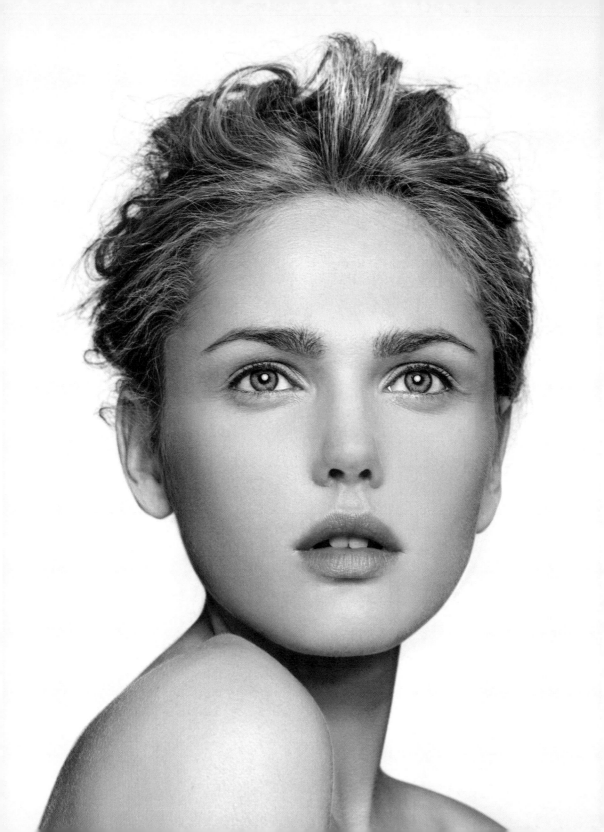

"The deepest part of a person is the skin"

Paul Valéry

The skin is by far the most extensive and the heaviest organ in the human body. The average adult skin consists of some two billion cells, has a surface area of 1.5-2 square meters (16- 21 square feet) and weighs 3-5 kilograms (7- 11 pounds) ...

But, remembering that we are essentially made of water, skin's most important role is as the barrier that maintains the body's water reserves. Water accounts for a hefty 60-70 per cent of our total body weight, 75 per cent at birth. In fact, our cells are so awash with H_2O that Gérard Redziniak, our scientific consultant in dermocosmetology, actually refers to human beings as "walking aquariums." On a more somber note, we can see why dehydration can be a life-threatening complication of third degree (widespread) burns.

The skin is also a sense organ, or should we say a sensor receptor organ, which interacts with the brain in extraordinarily subtle ways. Scientists have demonstrated that severely premature babies are significantly more likely to survive if they are massaged every day. Quite apart from its benefits for the respiratory system, massage is believed to reinforce the skin's role as an antimicrobial barrier, and also serves to prevent dehydration and weight loss.

Those interactions between body, mind and spirit are at the heart of everything we do at Cinq Mondes. Our spa therapists cultivate the art of touch in all of its infinite complexity, using therapies and petroleum-free cosmetics that build up natural skin thanks to ultra-pure, high-fat plant oils that feed the skin with Omega 3, 6 and 9 essential fatty acids. For comparison, silicones and mineral oils are used in some 80 per cent of all beauty products, but they have no physical or chemical affinity whatsoever with skin.

CELL HOMEOSTASIS:
A DELICATE BALANCE

The objective is to restore the skin's natural balance, or what is known as homeostasis – from *homeios* (the same) and *stasis* (staying). Well-balanced skin is healthy skin, and it is the mission of modern cosmetic science to promote that balance. This it does through skincare products that address the needs of the "whole person," reflecting the view of health as defined by the WHO in 1948: "a state of complete physical, mental and social wellbeing and not merely the absence of disease or infirmity."

Restoring cell homeostasis is one of the major challenges facing cosmetics research, focusing on protecting the skin from environmental factors, and protecting the human genome from the exposome (the sum total of the factors that threaten cellular equilibrium).

An incredible machine

Skin is naturally built for strength, with a structure like a house, complete with roof, frame and brickwork. The epidermis is the roof, composed of tile-like stem cells that extend upwards from the basal layer to the superficial corneal epithelium (Latin for "horny layer"), where they become flattened, losing their nuclei but remaining biochemically active. The intercellular cement is the frame, composed of substances such as lipids and ceramides; and the keratinocytes are the bricks, consisting of some 1,800 billion cells with a roughly cuboid shape.

When working as nature intended, the human skin is a perfectly balanced system. Every cell is a miniature chemical factory, capable of churning out 30,000 different products, from the simplest to the most complex molecules. Hundreds of millions of coordinated chemical reactions play out in the skin all the time, varying according to the body's needs – and we don't even know this is happening. So it is that a mountain of data is constantly decoded to

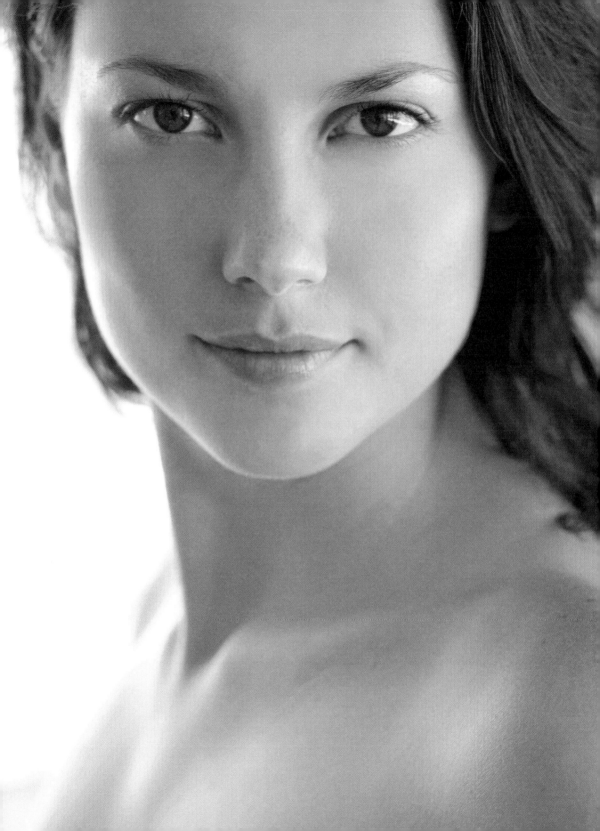

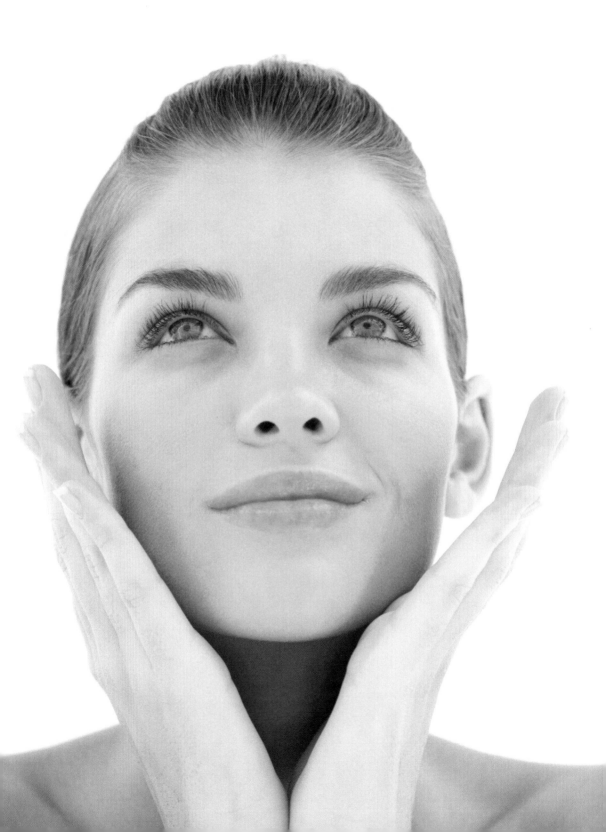

allow synthesis and assimilation, or on the contrary the decomposition of thousands of chemical substances in order to maintain optimal body functioning. It is worth remembering here that the human body is quite literally "born from dust" – composed of 26 chemical elements that are among the 92 elements or compounds present in the Earth's crust. The body constantly recreates itself from these elements. Every breath brings forth a new body, complete with everything required for its balanced functioning.

Every atom, every molecule in the body must be constantly renewed. The cells of the epidermis rejuvenate every three to four weeks. Colon cells meanwhile renew themselves every three to four days. Every minute, 200 million cells die and 200 million new cells take over. It is this capacity for auto-regeneration that makes tissue donation possible: after donating blood or bone marrow your body replaces all of the cells that have been lost. Every second indeed, 2-3 million RBCs (red blood cells) are produced in the bone marrow – that's 200 billion RBCs per day.

Factors that threaten balance

The problem is that our modern lifestyle disrupts homeostasis due to environmental hazards known collectively as the exposome.

One of the biggest threats to homeostasis is excessive exposure to UVA and UVB but also blue light, particularly from computer and TV screens. UVB increases epidermal thickness by stimulating cell proliferation at the outermost layer of skin. UVA meanwhile "breaks" the double-helix structure of DNA, reducing skin elasticity and producing wrinkles. Even in town, the incidence of UVB-induced photo-aging is quite dramatic. Your average 65-year old taxi driver will typically look 20 years older on the curbside of his face than on the cab side. Exposure to blue (screen) light has the same effect.

Pollution is another factor that jeopardizes homeostasis and contributes to premature skin aging. In town, tiny airborne particles produced by combustion (chimneys, exhaust systems, cigarettes) pose a constant threat to our wellbeing (in the country you have pesticides and herbicides to worry about). The culprit is benzo[a]pyrene, a molecule generated by combustion that is detected by the aryl hydrocarbon receptor in the skin. Known as the AhR, this functions as a "sensor" that recognizes danger signals such as pollutants and triggers a cellular inflammatory response. The result is chronic, low-grade inflammation or what we now call "inflammaging:" a major factor in premature aging because it induces the production of volatile free radicals that cause oxidative damage. These free radicals eat away at cells walls making "holes" – what you might call "cell rusting."

The skin also has to fend off pollutants such as greenhouse gases, including the ozone (O_3) emissions produced by the combined effects of carbon dioxide and solar radiation on exhaust systems.

Loss of homeostasis

A third factor that disrupts cell homeostasis is psychological stress. When the body feels tense or anxious, it releases cortisol (aka the aging hormone), a naturally occurring glucocorticoid that serves to improve performance. When the immediate stress is over, the levels of cortisol dissipate. At times, however, cortisol levels remain elevated due to repetitive exposure to stress or the slow dissipation of cortisol, as recorded in post-menopausal women. When that happens, the skin's ability to regenerate is impaired, homeostasis fails and the immune system is weakened. The Langerhans cells among the keratinocytes can no longer do their job properly, which is to engulf antigens and steer them toward the death-dealing lymphocytes.

Another factor in skin aging is smoking. Cigarette smoke is packed with extremely aggressive particles, called free radicals, which oxidize (rust) the cells. Less well known, perhaps, is the fact that inhaling cigarette smoke indirectly prevents the protection of elastin (a highly elastic protein that makes the skin supple) via inhibition

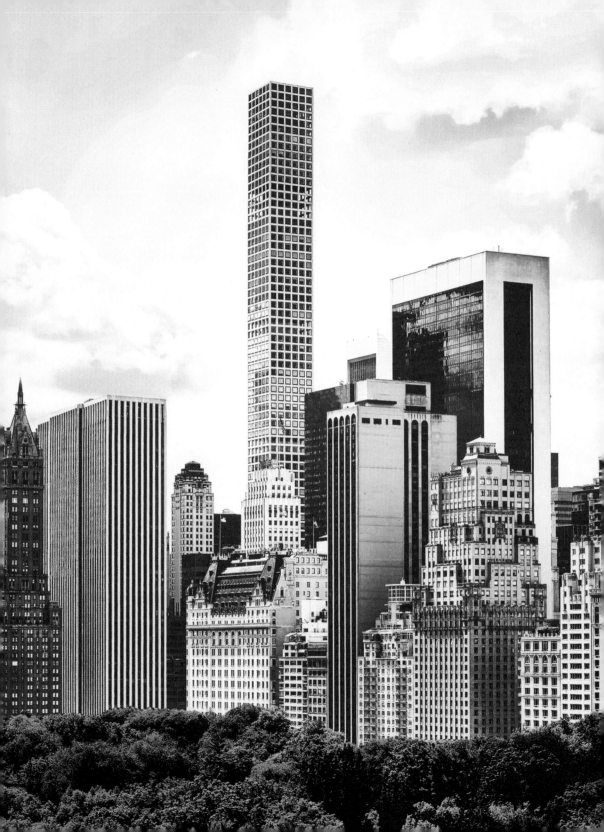

of an enzyme called elastase. This is because elastin decomposition is related to elastase activity, which is inhibited by a protein produced in the liver called Alpha1-Antitrypsin (AAT). Smoking is known to accelerate1 Alpha1-Antitrypsin deficiency, increasing elastase activity, with an attendant loss of tissue elasticity.

Elastin ensures the structural integrity and recoil capacity of the skin. Collagen meanwhile provides the skin with the resilience it needs to withstand stretching. When you consider that it takes 70 and 15 years respectively for elastin and collagen fibers to renew themselves, it is easy to see why smoking causes wrinkles. Not long ago I saw a photo of twin sisters now in their seventies, one a smoker for 40 years, the other a non-smoker. The difference between them was striking – they hardly looked like sisters, never mind twins.

Endocrine disruptors

Last but not least, there are endocrine disruptors: the hormonal effects of every-day toxins and the challenges they pose for public health authorities. Hundreds of endocrine disruptors exist in household goods including … cosmetics! Endocrine disrupting chemicals (EDCs) are divided into two groups: EDCs that affect steroid action (interfering with the reproductive system); and EDCs that affect thyroid hormone activity (interfering with the body's ability to maintain a constant core temperature). What makes EDCs particularly worrying is that they challenge one of the basic principles of toxicology, as expressed in Paracelsus' famous maxim: "All things are poison and nothing is without poison; only the dose makes a thing not a poison."

In fact, a single high-dose exposure to EDCs poses no systemic risk because their effects are detected and neutralized by the body's defense mechanisms. Chronic, low-dose exposure is another matter entirely. The effects are particularly insidious because a) they are not immediately apparent (and may even be passed down to future generations); and b) they cannot be studied in isolation. In other words, the effect of each individual substance cannot be isolated from the combined effect – what's known as the "cocktail effect".

There is now evidence that the endocrine disrupting effects of pesticides, herbicides, estrogens (the pill in particular) and phytoestrogens (eg in soya milk) can actually cause sex changes in fish. I heard this from a scientist in Brittany who informed me that there are so few male fish left in the Bay of Quiberon that the authorities have had to resort to reintroduction programs.

As mentioned earlier, many of the ingredients now in the dock are contained in cosmetics – typically, parabens, phthalates and alkylphenols – but very little information exists about their impact. All the more reason, therefore, for those of us working in cosmetics to be particularly vigilant about the safety of our own products. Indeed, we shall see that petroleum-free cosmetics that sooth, repair and rebuild skin can be quite remarkably effective in the battle against "environmental aggressors" – especially when accompanied by lifestyle changes.

" Petrochemicals are also a public health concern "

These are the products that we make at Cinq Mondes – new-generation cosmetics that resolutely part company with their industrially made counterparts. Instead of silicones and mineral oils that clog skin pores (present in some 80 per cent of the beauty products on this planet) we use rare and precious plant oils that heal, repair and draw on intelligent thinking to combat environmental aggressors. True, our ingredients cost a lot more – 150 euros a kilo compared to just eight for silicones and mineral oils – but then price is not an issue for us, as it is for conventional producers. Actually the jasmine absolute in our Crème Riche de Jeunesse costs an eye-watering 9,000 euros a kilo – expensive certainly, but considering its exceptional phyto-aromatic benefits, well worth the money.

REDISCOVERING
THE LOST PARADISE
OF HOMEOSTASIS

You could of course argue that we are not all created equal in terms of skin aging. Genetic factors do certainly play a part in the rate at which our cells age. But with advances in epigenetics (the science that studies the impact of lifestyle factors on ... genetics itself) we are gradually coming to understand how the exposome eventually imprints itself in our genome over the course of our lives.

High exposure to exposomal factors leads to an insidious weakening of our genetic heritage. But epigenetics shows that the reverse is also true. Rethinking our lifestyles, minimizing sun exposure and exposure to pollution and tobacco smoke, can have a positive effect on our genetic heritage.

In fact balanced living, together with appropriate skin care products, are our two key weapons in the fight against toxic substances – even in cities where EDCs are all around us.

CHANGING
THE WAY WE LIVE

Balanced living, changing our habits for better health, is something we have been studying for years at Cinq Mondes. To make that change, we need to rethink five aspects of our everyday lives. One: we must learn to eat for health and pleasure. Two: we must rediscover restful sleep with relaxing bedtime rituals. Three: we must adapt our daily routine to include simple, energizing exercises – yoga or Qi Gong for instance. Four: we must take better care of our bodies through massage and self-massage. And Five, we must make time for the health benefits of water (baths, Turkish baths, swimming ...).

At Cinq Mondes we have explored each of these five dimensions in detail, drawing on the knowledge of physicians from different walks of life in order to offer enriching experiences that may now be enjoyed at our "Spa and Wellness Retreats." It's an entirely new concept in spa care: a holistic approach to wellness that considers the whole person, within a retreat-like setting that shakes up old habits. For many people, escaping from it all for a few days is like pressing the reset button on their lives.

Today, in 2018, there are three such retreats on our Cinq Mondes "planet". One is at the Beau Rivage Palace in Lausanne: the ideal place for a restorative stay in superb natural surroundings, complete with an Anne Sophie Pic gourmet restaurant and our 1500m2 (16000sq ft) Cinq Mondes spa. One is at the Long Beach Tropical Resort in Mauritius: a tropical paradise featuring a 2000m2 (21,500 sq ft) Cinq Mondes spa with everything you need for a head-to-toe rescue. And one is at the Kempinski Emerald Palace in Palm Jumeirah, Dubaï: 3000m2 (32,000sq ft) of spa facilities (making this the largest Cinq Mondes spa in the world) with 30 treatment rooms, plus eight villas each with its own 250m2 (2,700 sq ft) private Cinq Mondes spa. Where better than these sensational surroundings to take stock of your life, with all the time you need to slough off old habits and make a fresh start.

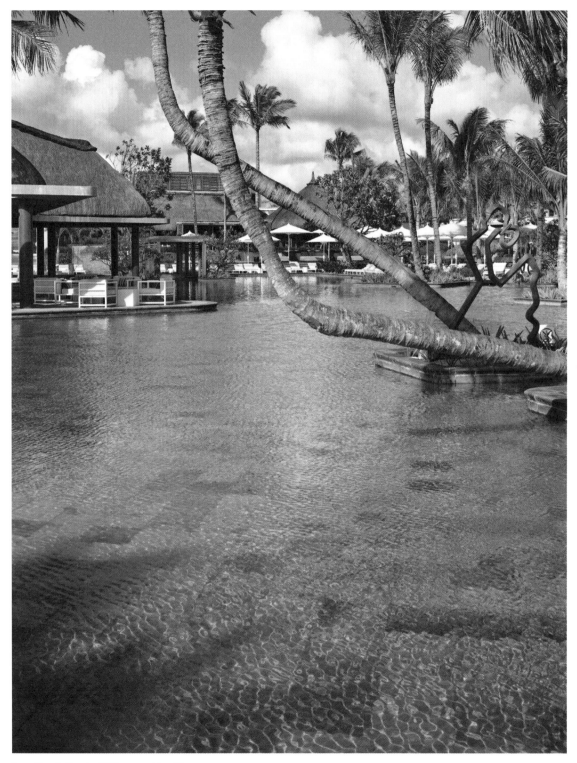

Long Beach Hotel, a SUN resort, Mauritius

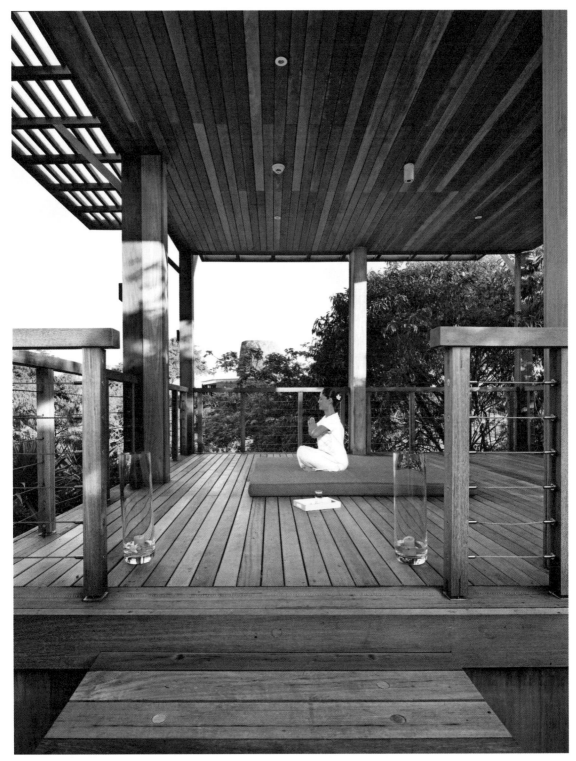

Yoga deck at Long Beach Hotel Cinq Mondes Spa, Mauritius

CINQ MONDES RETREATS ARE FOUNDED ON FIVE BASIC PILLARS OF HEALTH

- 1 -

Good nutrition, focusing on specially selected detox juices and recipes, plus healthy eating habits. For example: always take the time to savor your food, not gulp it down. Because we know that eating slowly is essential for good digestion, there are egg timers on all of the tables in our Spa and Wellness Retreats restaurants. It's an invitation to slow down, eat mindfully, cultivate a new approach to eating. Slow eating makes for better digestion, which is definitely a key factor in regulating our bodily processes on a daily basis.

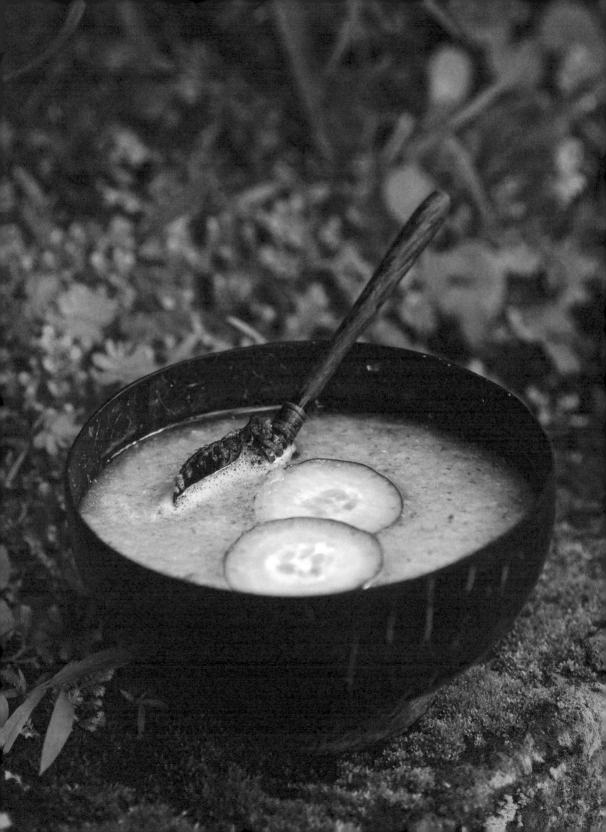

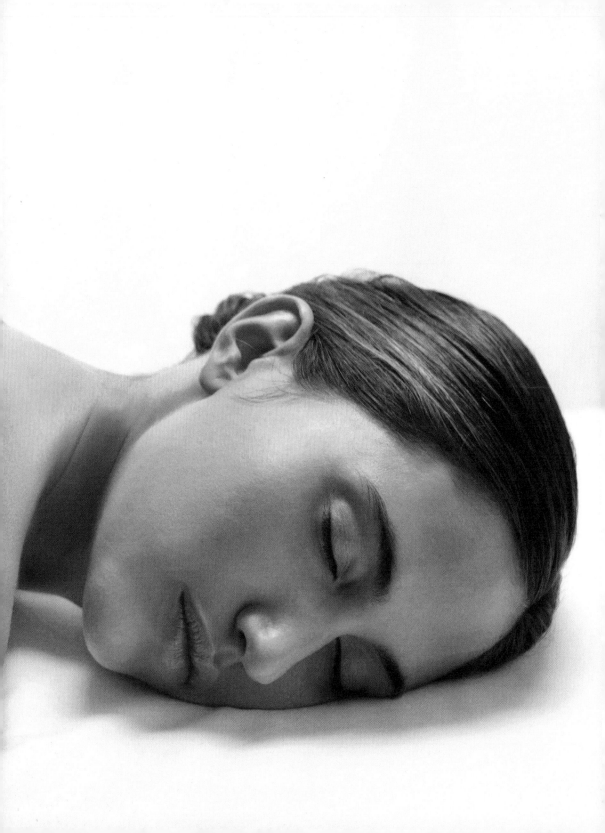

Pillar Number Two: Good quality sleep to repair and restore the mind and body. Our treatments for bedtime are specifically designed to promote a good night's sleep. They include Ayurvedic Sirodhara therapy: drizzling warm sesame oil in a continuous stream between the temples to induce a deep, trance-like state of relaxation. We also provide encouragements to wind down before bed – such as offering a choice of pillows to ensure the best possible sleeping posture. And to perfect your bedtime rituals, our Cinq Mondes pillow mist brings you soothing fragrances to lull you into slumber: Eau Egyptienne, a sleep potion combining 11 essential oils that Queen Hatshepsut Pharaoh of Egypt used as perfume, described by Plutarch as "allaying anxieties and brightening dreams."

3

Pillar Number Three: Spa therapy (naturally), based on three kinds of health program lasting from three to five days or longer:

• **An Ayurvedic health program** to rebalance the doshas and purify body and mind through a variety of tried and trusted treatments such as Abhyanga, Kansu and Sirodhara.

• **A Taoist health program** inspired by the time-honored principles of *Tui Na* massage (Chinese Therapeutic Massage) and foot reflexology, plus the rebalancing of Qi (vital energy) using the Chinese medicine five-elements theory.

• **A detox program,** complete with cleansing and lymphatic drainage treatments such as Udarabhyanga and especially Urdvartana – a specialized Ayurveda treatment for effective weight loss that involves kneading, friction, vibration and percussion movements, combined with the power of traditional herbal remedies (ginger, *Emblica officinalis* and garbanzos bean flour to drain the fluids and toxins that can build up in the tissues ...)

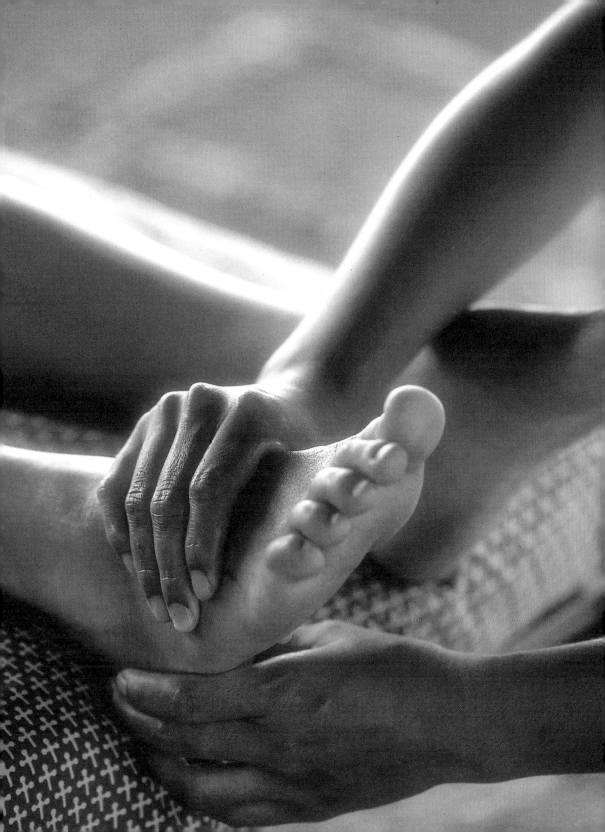

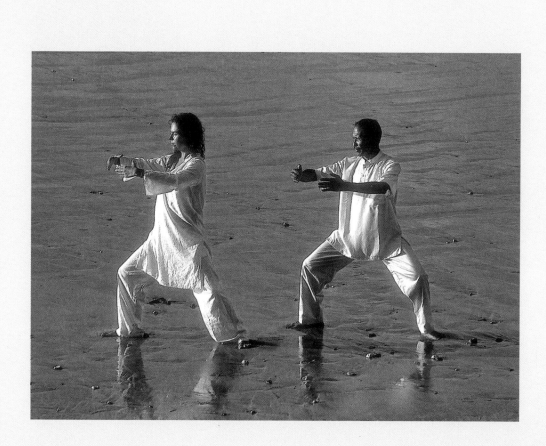

4

Pillar Number Four: Yoga and Qi Gong exercises to boost energy and improve flexibility. Harnessing the breath through daily practice allows us to access our life-force energy, rebalancing body and mind and bringing renewed vitality together with a profound sense of relaxation. The word *yoga* in Sanskrit means "union" and has come to mean a method for mastering prana, the life force. Asanas (poses) and breathing techniques establish the framework for practice, which brings benefits from the very first sessions. Yoga as a way of life has always been an integral part of Ayurveda. Likewise Qi Gong, from Qi "vital life energy" and Gong "effort and discipline", focuses on soft, flowing movements that work to reinforce and purify life energy, harmonize the flow of Qi for long life and physical and mental wellbeing. Qi Gong is one of the Five Pillars of Traditional Chinese Medicine and promotes letting-go, serenity and creativity.

5

Pillar Number Five: Water – because spas and water have always been inseparable (some claim that the word spa is an acronym of the Latin phrase *sanitas per aquam* meaning "health through water"). Water is the medium that surrounds our first nine months and the element to which we are instinctively drawn thereafter to cleanse the mind and body. So the fifth pillar of our retreats naturally consists of different forms of hydrotherapy. Among these, our aromatic and color therapy Turkish bath combines the benefits of steam at 45 degrees Celsius (about 110 degrees Fahrenheit), with Five Element aromatherapy, and cromatherapy as defined in our Cinq Mondes "Aroma and Color Wheel." Other highlights include our traditional Japanese aromatic bath sprinkled with flower petals (ofuro) – a whole art and ritual in itself, cleansing the heart and flushing out toxins – and tubs with water at just the right temperature to immerse your body in bliss, pounded by massage jets of healing water.

These five pillars of health create the right conditions for a return to health and vitality while also inducing a deep state of relaxation and inner peace that brings untold blessings. As the endocrine system steps up release of your happy hormones (oxytocins, endorphins...), the attendant reduction in cortisol (stress hormone) levels helps to prevent the oxidative stress, or cell rusting, which causes the skin to age at the cellular level. And when that happens, happiness can indeed be said to come from the skin!

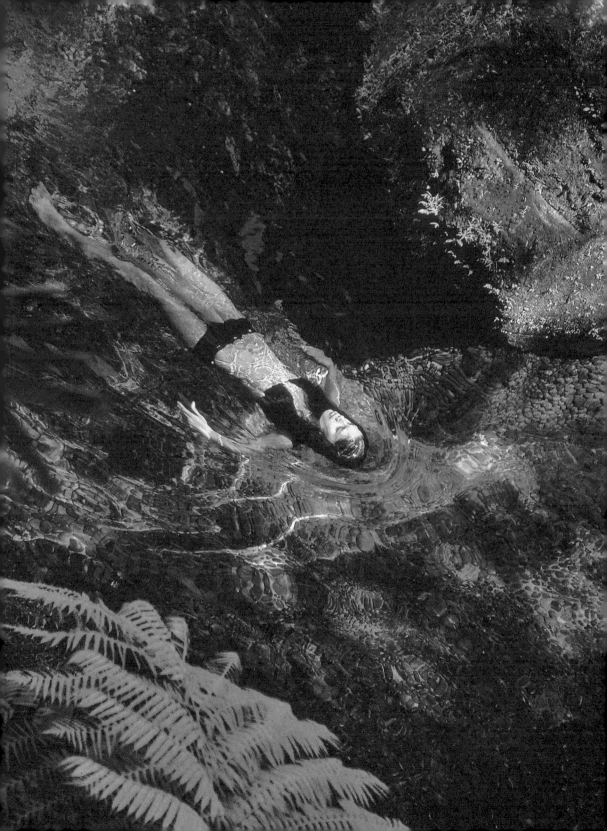

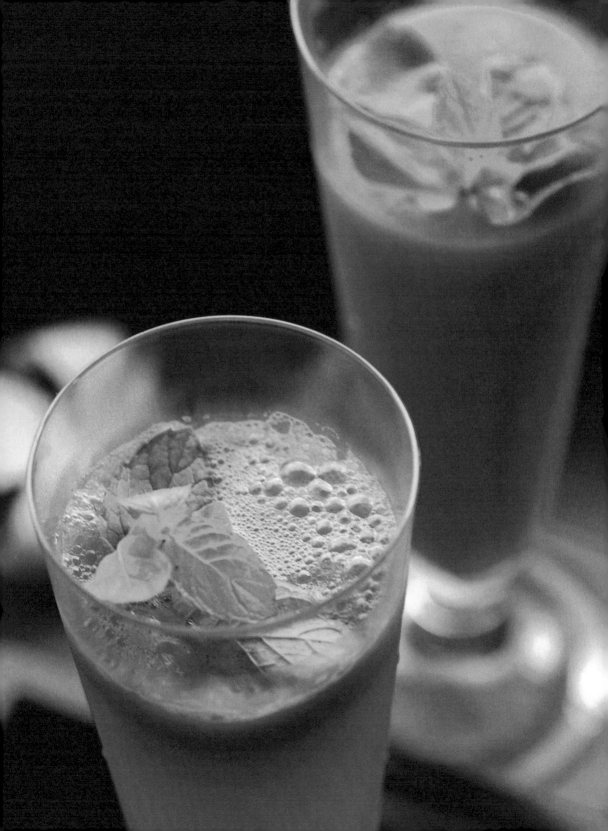

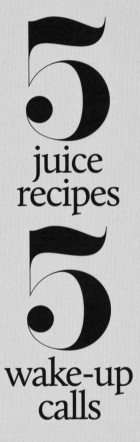

5
juice
recipes

5
wake-up
calls

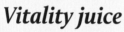

2

Wake-up to
the joy of commitment

Citrus and carrot energizer

INGREDIENTS
½ GRAPEFRUIT
1½ ORANGES
1½ CARROTS

Peel and chop the fruit, wash the carrot, then place all the ingredients in the juicer/blender. Add another carrot if necessary to counter the sharpness of the grapefruit.

Drink freshly made, soon after juicing.

1

Wake-up to
the joy of self-betterment

Vitality juice

INGREDIENTS
20CL/7FL OZ COCONUT WATER
1 ORANGE
2 HANDFULS SPINACH
125G/4OZ MANGO
FEW DROPS LEMON JUICE

Peel and chop the fruit then place all the ingredients in a juicer/blender and process until smooth. Add more fruit or coconut water depending on how thick or thin you like your smoothies.

3

Wake-up to
the joy of letting go

Orange and fennel relaxer

INGREDIENTS
2 ORANGES (OR 150ML/5 FL OZ ORANGE JUICE)
1TBS BROWN SUGAR
½ TSP CINNAMON POWDER
1 MEDIUM SIZE FENNEL BULB CHOPPED

Peel the oranges then place in the juicer with the oranges, fennel, brown sugar and cinnamon. Process until smooth and enjoy right away.

---

*Wake-up to the joy
of the present moment*

Vegetable and fruit comforter

INGREDIENTS
3 CARROTS
1 BEET
1 APPLE
2 BRANCHES CELERY
½ CUCUMBER
½ GLASS OF WATER
OR 100ML/4FL OZ COCONUT WATER
HANDFUL ICE CUBES (OPTIONAL)

Begin by washing the vegetables and fruit thoroughly to remove any bacteria. Then cut into small dice and place in the juicer, adding the water or coconut juice to make processing easier plus the ice cubes according to taste.

———

*Wake-up to the joy
of intellectual creativity*

Lemony pepper and cucumber illuminator

INGREDIENTS
1 LEMON
½ BELL PEPPER
¼ CUCUMBER
1 CARDAMOM POD
1TBS RADISH OR OTHER BEAN SPROUTS
(AVAILABLE FROM ALL GOOD HEALTH FOOD SHOPS)

Peel the lemon, wash the vegetables then split open the cardamom pod and scrape out five seeds. Place all the ingredients in the juicer/blender and process until smooth. Drink chilled.

———

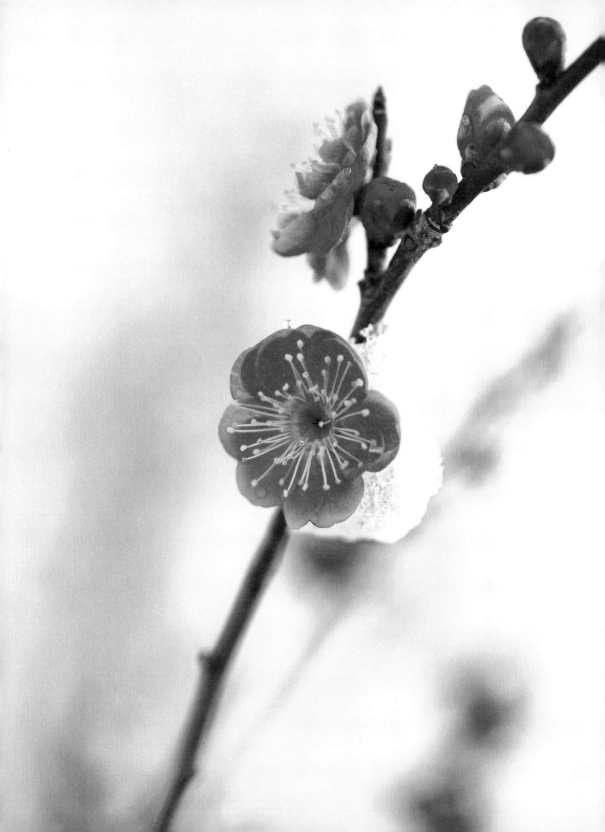

PROTECTING
AND REGENERATING
YOUR SKIN

It is of course essential to restore the fundamental balance of our mind-body complex, and our five pillars of health embody a preventive approach that is designed to do just that. But skin care is equally important: the application of cosmetic products that are absorbed through the skin, helping to balance and stimulate cell metabolism by offering protection against the skin-aging exposome and free radical damage.

As we saw earlier, the petroleum-based cosmetics produced by the big conventional beauty brands have no affinity with skin and are not good for the skin. Mineral oils and silicones represent some 99 per cent of their composition. The remaining one per cent consists of plant extracts (rose, cornflower, burdock or some other plant extract) that are blatantly exploited by all of these companies to promote their products as "plant-based."

At Cinq Mondes, we offer products based on own unique formulae that bring real benefits to the skin. Products composed of 100 per cent plant oils, rich in essential fatty acids, vitamins and antioxidants, with powerful tissue regenerative and wound healing properties ...

The power of Omega 3, 6 and 9 essential fatty acids

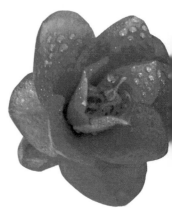

Our Élixirs Précieux are thus exclusively composed of "ultra-pure plant oils" such as argan, kemiri and camellia oil. Bursting with fatty acids, they work to reinforce the skin barrier, regulate moisture levels, prevent inflammation, promote wound healing and ward off free radical attacks. They are specifically designed to preserve the acid mantle that keeps the skin looking young.

Omega 3 fatty acids have anti-inflammatory properties that make them a natural choice in the making of soothing skincare products. They are also excellent emollients (skin softeners).

Omega 6 fatty acids consist essentially of linoleic acid. They also play a role in the barrier function of the skin, but are particularly interesting for their effects on skin elasticity.

Omega 9 fatty acids consist essentially of oleic acid, which is not strictly "essential" (meaning it can be produced by the body). Omega 9 fatty acids are nevertheless all important dietary fats (even found in human sebum) and interesting for their effects on skin hydration, protection, suppleness and elasticity.

Vitamins and antioxidants

Antioxidants are another very interesting group of substances. They serve to neutralize the free radicals that are mainly created by the cells of the immune system, and which are actually not all bad because they contribute to the proper functioning of cells. The problems start when they increase uncontrollably, which as we have seen is more likely to happen in smokers and sun worshippers, and in times of physical or psychological stress. When produced in excess, free radicals accelerate skin aging.

So to make sure your skin gets plenty of antioxidants, like beta-carotene (Vitamin A) and Vitamins C and E, you have to eat the right foods and apply the right skin care. The best dietary sources are fruit, vegetables and legumes (beans). The best topical sources are skincare products containing a cocktail of high-performance ingredients – as found in our Sérum Lumière Sublime Cinq Mondes. This concentrated antioxidant and dark spot ("age spot") corrector serum boasts essential ingredients from carefully sourced plants that are known for their high vitamin content: Vitamin B and C plus bioflavonoids from the goji berries of the Lycium Chinense, a shrub native to

Japan; Vitamin E and Omega 9 fatty acids from Japanese rose oil, to regulate the keratinization of epidermal cells and protect them; and rutin (Vitamin P), from the flower buds of the Sophora Japonica or Japanese pagoda tree, a bioflavonoid whose powerful anti-inflammatory effects help to combat inflammaging.

But vitamins are not the only effective antioxidants ... Our Sérum Lumière Sublime Cinq Mondes also contains a compound made from *Magnolia kobus* (closely related to *Magnolia stellata* or "star magnolia") and *Glycyrrhiza glabra* (licorice), which have been clinically proven to be one hundred times more effective than Vitamin C.

Nature thus offers a treasure trove of plants and substances that are inherently more effective than synthetic preparations and petroleum-based substances!

I cannot resist here including a historical anecdote about Vitamin C. The chemical name for Vitamin C is ascorbic acid, which comes from the Latin scorbutus: a severe Vitamin C deficiency caused by the absence of fresh fruit and vegetables. Better known as scurvy, the disease is deadly if untreated and remained the scourge of seafarers right up until the 19th century. Its most telltale symptom was loss of teeth, Vitamin C being essential to the production of collagen, the substance that holds the body together!

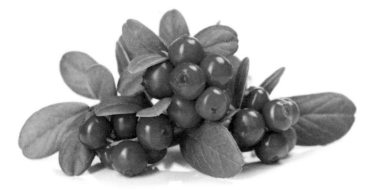

Uvaxine, from Japanese knotweed

The origin of this active ingredient is a story that deserves to be told because it illustrates the genius of nature – and of the man who managed to discover it.

The man in question was Gérard Redziniak, a PhD in molecular biophysiochemistry and our scientific consultant in cosmetics innovation. It is thanks to him that Uvaxcine now ranks among the proprietary ingredients in our Sérum Lumière Sublime. Because Gérard Redziniak is not so much an inventor as a "cosmetological humanist" – a man so dedicated to human ecology that he prefers to "teach cells to defend themselves", not cover them with chemical sunscreens that block UVA and UVB. As he rightly points out, "Give a man a fish and you feed him for a day. Teach a man to fish and you feed him for a lifetime."

Uvaxine is an active ingredient obtained by enzymatic synthesis of a protein in Japanese knotweed, a medicinal herb cultivated throughout Asia. Among other things, Uvaxine acts as a stimulator of Nrf2: a key signaling protein that triggers the expression of antioxidant genes at times of free radical or UV-induced toxic stress. Uvaxine has the potential to augment Nrf2 activity and facilitate its accumulation, giving it a preventive mode of action. In this respect, it works rather like a vaccine – hence its name, Uvaxine.

Our Sérum Lumière Sublime Cinq Mondes combines Uvaxine with Vitamins B, C, E, P and the compound *Magnolia kobus*-licorice, offering a mix of natural ingredients with an incredibly complex mode of action. That's what I love about scientific research: the endless affinities between plants and skin never cease to amaze me!

Plant stem cells

Stem cells are another miracle of biology: undifferentiated cells that can self-renew (make more stem cells) and differentiate into specialized cells. They are contained in our Crème Précieuse Nuit Cinq Mondes in the form of "cellulosomes": multicomponent complexes obtained from sea holly (*Eryngium Maritimum*), a halophytic plant that is supremely adapted to very saline soils but also does well under normal conditions. More precisely, cellulosomes are multi-enzyme and plant stem cell machines for degradation that improve the uptake of nutrients. Their action enhances the bioavailability of skincare products, occurring within cells at a key moment in chronobiology – nighttime – when microcirculation and cell division peak. This allows the regeneration and renewal of basal keratinocytes; the restructuring of the derma-epidermal junction; and the reduction of light-induced inflammation. To put it simply, these stem cells make it possible to stimulate cell regeneration and improve the architecture of the dermis. Which is about as far as you can get from the "plastic wrap effect" you get with silicone and mineral oil based industrial cosmetics.

Peptides

Continuing on the theme of Nature's infinite wisdom, let us now turn to the peptides contained in our Crème Précieuse Cinq Mondes.

Peptides are short chains of amino acids that play a messenger role between cells and also act as neurotransmitters. Peptides send signals to the skin cells, triggering more collagen production when certain proteins or major components in the skin matrix and derma-epidermal junction have been damaged (for instance collagen types 1, 3 and 4, fibronectin and laminin 5). Peptides thus make it possible to restart natural processes and regenerate those skin cells most in need of repair ...

In short, these little marvels of Nature are a further reason to place our trust in a subtle understanding of cell biology and not petrochemical technologies!

Hyaluronic acid

To complete our tour of the wonderworks in Nature's skin-boosting arsenal, there is hyaluronic acid: the greatest water-holding champion of them all, with unparalleled ability to hydrate the skin. Hyaluronic acid, or to be more precise, botanical hyaluronic acid, is obtained from fermentation of lactic bacteria adapted to a wheat substrate. It is what's known as a biomimetic ingredient, meaning it mimics natural biological mechanisms – hence its ability to develop a perfect affinity with skin. When applied topically, it prevents water loss and shields the skin from external aggressors, binding up to one thousand times its own molecular weight in water. Hyaluronic acid is Nature's "moisture magnet", invaluable in the fight against dehydration wrinkles!

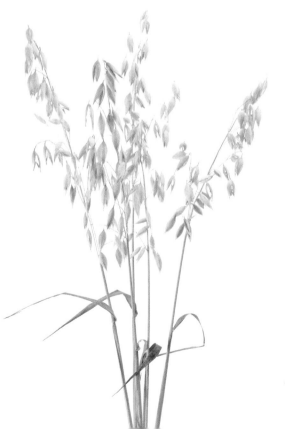

Cinq Mondes
"Crème Riche de Jeunesse"

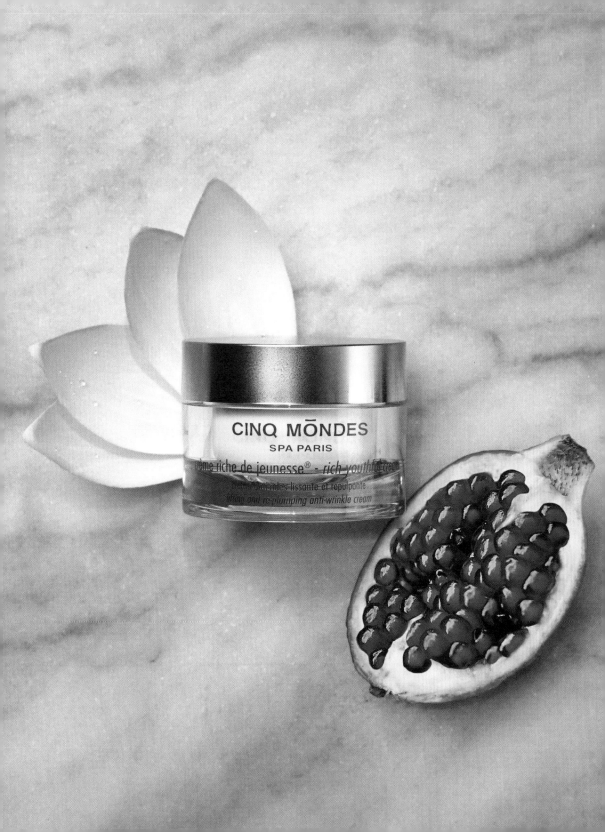

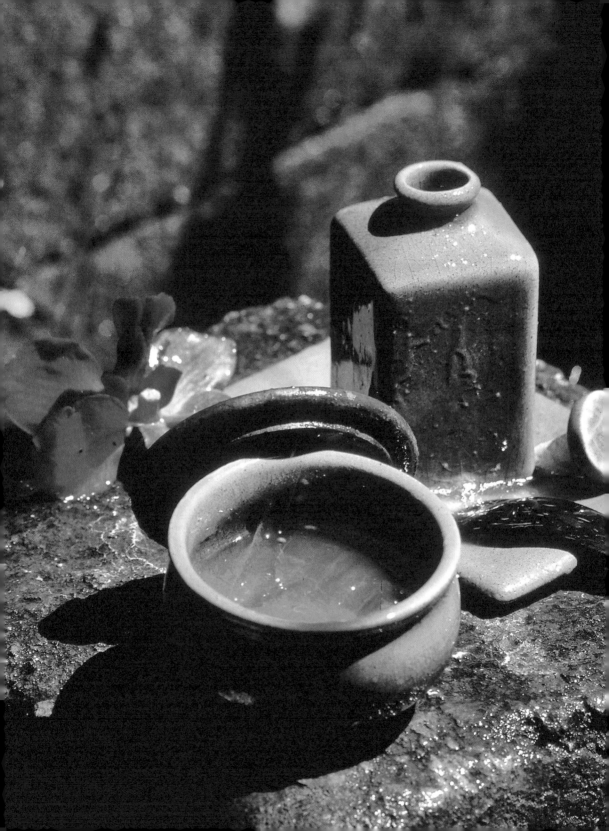

BEAUTY RECIPES
INSPIRED BY ANCIENT RITUALS FOR YOU TO TRY AT HOME

Let yourself be inspired by beauty recipes gleaned from
the greatest cultural traditions. Become your very own
"beauty chef". Gather together the ingredients then wash
your hands and all utensils and prepare to enjoy yourself.
Do remember to keep these goodies in the icebox
and use within a week.

1

Fights tiredness, adds instant glow and regulates sebum production, giving you a healthy, radiant complexion.

PURIFYING AND BALANCING MASK

INSPIRED BY A TRADITIONAL RECIPE FROM ANCIENT SYRIA

INGREDIENTS
50G/4OZ KAOLIN
1TSP HENNA POWDER
½ TSP GRAPEFRUIT SEED EXTRACT
3 DROPS SAGE ESSENTIAL OIL
2 DROPS ROSEMARY ESSENTIAL OIL
WATER TO MIX

Mix with water to form a smooth paste and use immediately. Apply generously to damp skin once or twice a week and leave to work for three to five minutes depending on skin type.

———

2

To feed dry or dehydrated skin, suitable for use as a day and/or night cream and as a repair facial mask.

DEEPLY NOURISHING FACIAL PASTE

INSPIRED BY AN ANCIENT ORIENTAL RECIPE

INGREDIENTS
20ML/0.6FLOZ SESAME OIL
30G/1OZ AVOCADO
½TSP HONEY
10 DROPS MYRRH OIL

To use as a repair facial mask, apply generously and leave to work for five minutes, then remove any excess with a damp cotton pad.

Tip: in winter, dab lightly onto lips to ease dryness and soreness.

———

3

Use as a skin booster before the facial paste, or alternatively add to the paste at the last minute to enhance its effects.

PRECIOUS NOURISHING BEAUTY OIL

INSPIRED BY AN ANCIENT RECIPE FROM MOROCCO

INGREDIENTS
10ML/0.3FL OZ SAFFLOWER OIL
(A NATURAL REMEDY FOR DRY SKIN)
10ML/0.3FL OZ ARGAN OIL (LIQUID GOLD!)
½TSP BLACK CUMIN OIL
5 DROPS ROSE ESSENCE

Gently massage into the skin using circular movements. Protects and regenerates thirsty skin like nothing else.

———

4

To restore freshness and awaken the senses.

HARMONIZING AROMATIC WATER

INSPIRED BY AN INDIAN LEGEND :

about the eternal love between the Emperor Shah Jahan and his wife Mumtaz Mahal, literally "Chosen One of the Palace", one of the loveliest women of the Empire whose beauty was sung by poets far and wide.
Warm scents of vanilla and cardamom combine to create a fragrant potion that may be sprayed onto the body and hair and also the pillow.

INGREDIENTS
30ML/1 FL OZ ALCOHOL
10 CRUSHED CARDAMOM SEEDS
½ TSP VANILLA OIL

Leave the cardamom seeds to macerate in the alcohol for about ten days, then add the vanilla oil.
Filter and luxuriate in the fragrance ...

———

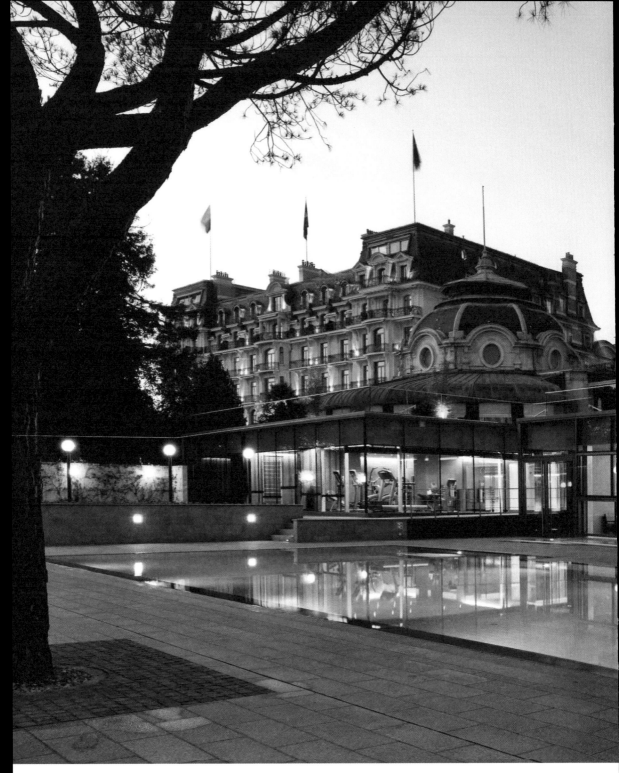

Cinq Mondes Spa at Beau Rivage Palace Hotel, Lausanne, Switzerland

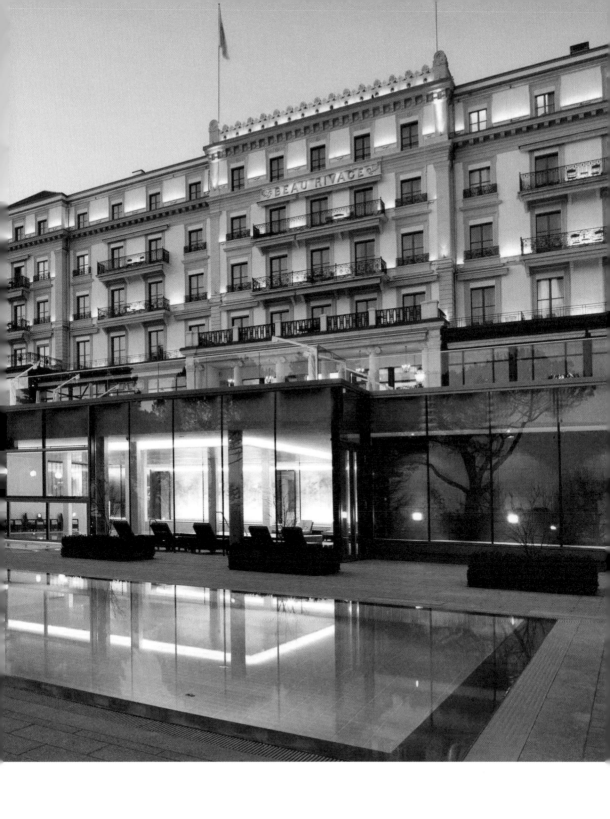

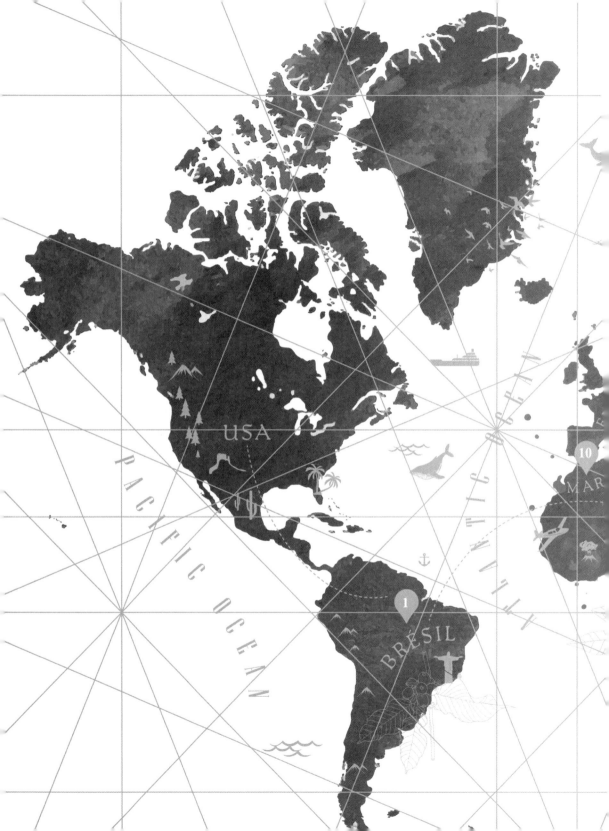

CONCLUSION

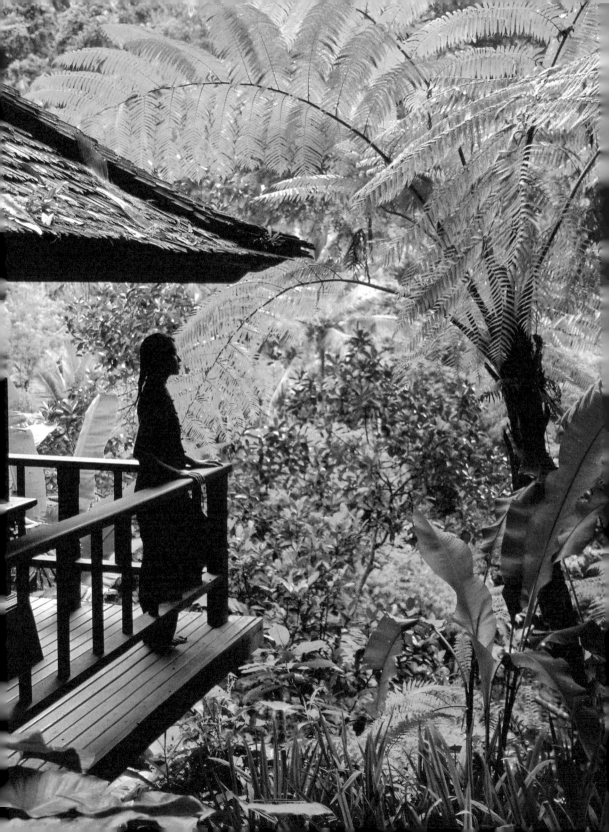

"Beauty is to me the Divine made visible, happiness made palpable, Heaven come down upon Earth."

THÉOPHILE GAUTIER,
MADEMOISELLE DE MAUPIN (1835)

I have enjoyed sharing my thoughts with you, looking at the concept "Happiness comes from the skin" and the many different meanings that I attach to it. As suggested by Théophile Gauthier in the above quotation, which I love, the links between wellbeing, beauty and happiness are actually much closer than rational thought might suggest.

My quest to understand these three qualities began with my discovery of Ayurveda in 1988 and has been gaining momentum ever since. In the course of those 30 years I have pursued a holistic vision of beauty that has led me to delve into cosmetics and traditional medicines and create an enterprise that could embody all the knowledge I had gained. The Cinq Mondes spa universe is the logical outcome of a lifetime's dedication to holistic wellbeing.

Those "Cinq Mondes" represent a distillation of all the skills and traditional healing practices of India, China, Japan, Siam and the Maghreb. But more than that, they span five different dimensions of the eternal quest for mind-body balance: that ideal state of equilibrium that can rejuvenate our whole being right down to the cellular level.

At Cinq Mondes I have the good fortune to be able to dedicate myself to five entirely complementary dimensions of wellness, beauty and health.

The first dimension is the creation of modern spaces that are essential to rejuvenate every aspect of our being, physically, psychologically, emotionally and even spiritually. Cinq Mondes spas are designed to do just that, drawing on creative thinking to provide tailor-made environments for the finest beauty rituals from around the world. Environments that bring together new approaches in lighting and materials design but also in chromotherapy, aromatherapy, Turkish baths, traditional Japanese baths – all of those therapies that enhance the experience of body and face massage.

The second dimension is the study of the remarkable benefits of what I call Cinq Mondes Dermapuncture: needle-free acupuncture based on age-old healing systems such as Ayurveda, Traditional Chinese Medicine (TCM) and shiatsu. All of these systems use the same acupressure points to stimulate and rebalance the metabolism, even though they all developed independently of each other, in different corners of the world and according to different theories. Proof if proof were needed that they are all firmly rooted in a profound and intimate understanding of the human being. The importance they attach to touch and massage is without parallel in Europe. The therapeutic effects of massage, mediated through touch, are considered key to balancing and stimulating the vital life force – what Ayurvedic practitioners call "prana" and TCM practitioners call "Qi". In every case the aim is to restore suppleness and energy to the body, the mind, and ultimately the skin.

The third dimension revolves around the fundamental role played by breathing and the art of breathing in the relief of stress: physical and emotional stress but also the oxidative stress associated with premature skin aging. And no-one knows better how important psycho-emotional balance is for youthful skin than Sri Sri Ravi Shankar, a world-renowned master of breath-work who I very much hope you will want to meet some day.

The fourth dimension relates to the extensive research we have conducted at Cinq Mondes, focusing on derma-cosmetology as the basis of what I call a Skin Nutrition Program: a science in its own right that aims to stimulate and rebalance cellular metabolism using proprietary plant ingredients that are shown to have affinities with the skin. These include, most notably, ten ultra-pure plant oils and 14 plant ingredients (all now patented Cinq Mondes technology). What they do not include are silicones and mineral oils that suffocate the skin, as still used today in 90 per cent of conventional cosmetics. All the more reason to make people aware that the skin interacts constantly with the body and the mind, that it is a living, breathing organ whose health is critical to our overall wellbeing.

The fifth dimension concerns my ongoing ethnography and botany "field trips", trying to understand the unique links between particular lifestyles and medicinal plants that are either consumed locally or included in cosmetic preparations. The lifestyle of the inhabitants of Okinawa in Japan is a good example. The island boasts the most centenarians per capita in the world and for three years now a Cinq Mondes team has been working with the islanders, documenting their way of life and the plants they use. What we have discovered is that they have a lot to teach us about healthy living. Okinawa residents live by the seasons and pace themselves accordingly. They live outdoors but stay in the shade as much as possible. They spend time with their families, live in a tight-knit community and exercise regularly. They also pursue their ikigaï: their reason for being, their purpose in life. For the Japanese, an ikigaï is anything that brings them joy – a dream, an ambition, an art – and it plays an important role in personal health and wellbeing. Many of the Okinawans also cultivate gardens where they grow wormwood (known for its anti-inflammatory and antimicrobial activity), ginger (which needs no introduction) and curcuma (a powerful anti-oxidant), plus an indigenous plant with remarkable anti-aging properties. Based on this ingredient, Cinq Mondes will soon launch a proprietary product that will mark an anti-aging breakthrough in the quest for youthful skin.

Because in the end, to draw inspiration from admirable lifestyles in far-flung places, from energizing practices that rework the mind and body and from advanced research on botany – these things are the real ingredients of a "happiness that comes from the skin."

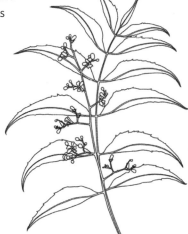

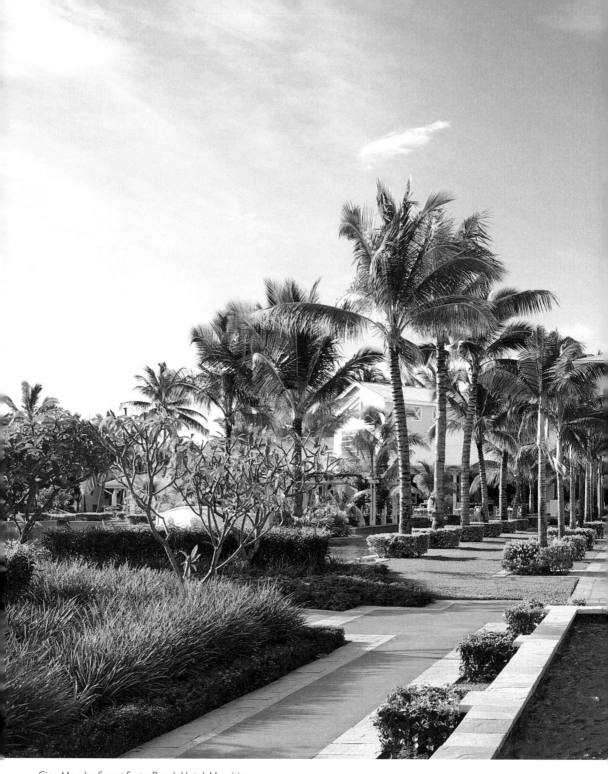

Cinq Mondes Spa at Sugar Beach Hotel, Mauritius

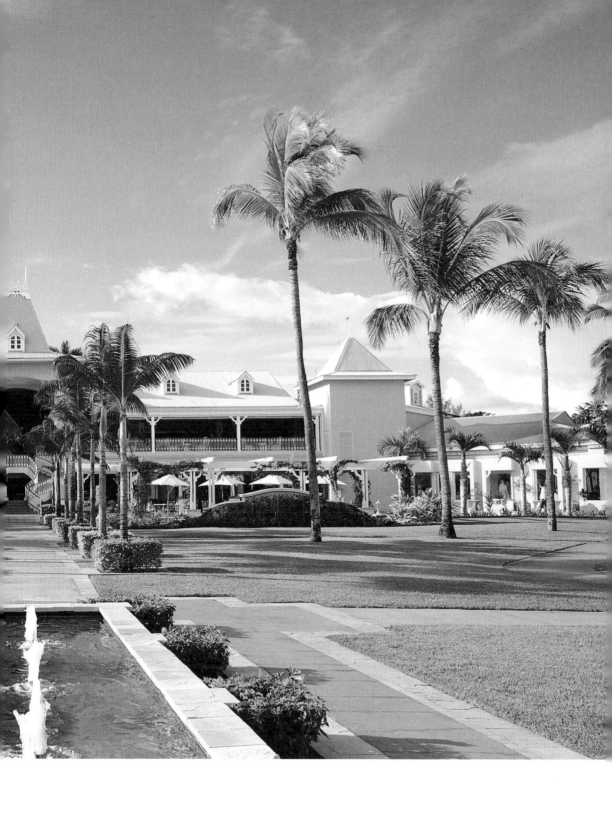

BIBLIOGRAPHY

Blackburn Elizabeth et Epel Elissa, *L'Effet télomère*, Guy Trédaniel éditeur, 2017.

Bouchon-Poiroux Nathalie et Ortéga Galya, *Massage ayurvédique*, Ellébore, 2015.

Clement Brian R. et DiGeronimo Theresa Foy, *Alimentation vivante pour une santé optimale*, Trustar, 1997.

Cohen Jean-Michel, *Qu'est-ce qu'on attend pour vivre mieux ?*, First, 2017.

Cusin Jacques-Pascal, *Les Secrets de l'alimentation vivante*, Albin Michel, 2012.

Enders Giulia, *Le Charme discret de l'intestin : tout sur un organe mal aimé*, Actes sud, 2015.

Foussier Valérie, *Perturbateurs endocriniens : ils sont partout ! Comment les éviter pour préserver sa santé*, Josette Lyon, 2017.

Guerven Estelle, *Biocosmétiques : la puissance de la nature au cœur de la beauté*, préface de Dominique Eraud, Guy Trédaniel éditeur, 2008.

Hämmerle Jean-François et Catz Clémence, *Les Plus Puissants des super-aliments*, Marabout, 2015.

Hampikian Sylvie, *Créez vos cosmétiques bio*, Terre vivante éditions, 2007.

Iyengar Bellur Krishnamachar Sundararaja, *Bible du yoga*, préface de Yehudi Menuhin, J'ai lu, 2009.

Laraison Émilie, *Encyclopédie des super aliments*, Flammarion, 2017.

Levesque Catherine, *Le Grand Livre antitoxique : perturbateurs endocriniens, additifs alimentaires, pesticides... se protéger de tous les poisons du quotidien*, LEDUC.S, 2017.

Marie Sophie et Tricot Lindsey, *Soin & beauté : mes recettes maison bio*, Saxe bien-être, 2017.

Michenaud Serge, *La Pratique de la respiration d'après l'enseignement de Sri Sri Ravi Shankar*, Le Courrier du livre, 2012.

Ortéga Galya et Poiroux Jean-Louis, *L'Art du bien-être dans le monde*, Aubanel, 2006.

Ortéga Galya et Poiroux Jean-Louis, *Massages et traditions chinoises*, Aubanel, 2009.

Ortéga Galya et Poiroux Jean-Louis, *Massages et traditions du Siam*, Aubanel, 2010.

Ortéga Galya et Poiroux Jean-Louis, *Massages et traditions indiennes*, Aubanel, 2009.

Ortéga Galya et Poiroux Jean-Louis, *Massages et traditions japonaises*, La Martinière, 2011.

Riveccio Patricia et Morfin Thierry, *Ma bible anti-perturbateurs endocriniens*, LEDUC.S, 2017.

Slama Rémy et Caro Denise, *Les Perturbateurs endocriniens : comment affectent-ils notre santé au quotidien ?*, éditions QUAE GIE, 2017.

Sonnenburg Justin, Sonnenburg Erica, *L'Incroyable Pouvoir du microbiote*, préface de Laurence Lévy-Dutel, 2017.

Sri Sri Ravi Shankar, *Celebrating Silence*, Art of Living Foundation, 2001.

Sri Sri Ravi Shankar, *Enseignements de l'art de vivre*, Dangles, 2003.

Sri Sri Ravi Shankar, *God Loves Fun*, The Art of Living, 1996.

Sri Sri Ravi Shankar, *Management Mantras*, Arktos, 2013.

Sri Sri Ravi Shankar, *Wisdom for the New Millenium*, Art of Living Foundation, 1999.

Van Lysebeth André et Herbert Jean, *J'apprends le yoga*, J'ai lu, 2004.

Yong Ed, *Moi, microbiote, maître du monde*, Dunod, 2017.

PHOTOGRAPHIC
CREDITS

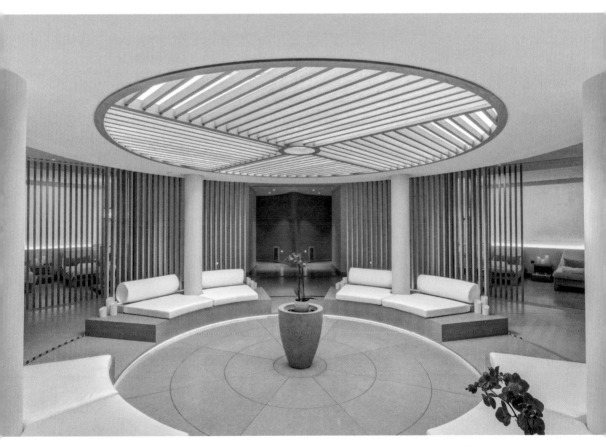

Cinq Mondes Spa at Monte Carlo Bay Hotel, Monaco

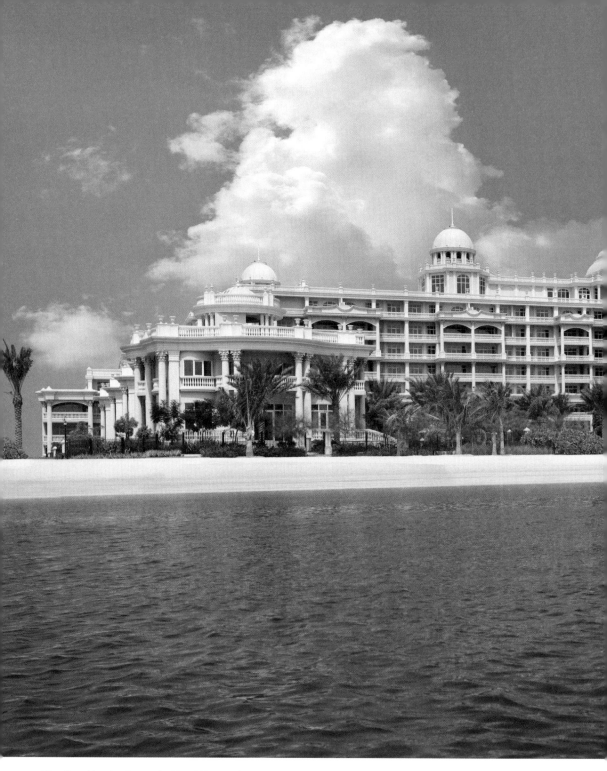

The Cinq Mondes Spa at the Hotel Kempinski, Palm Jumeirah, Dubai

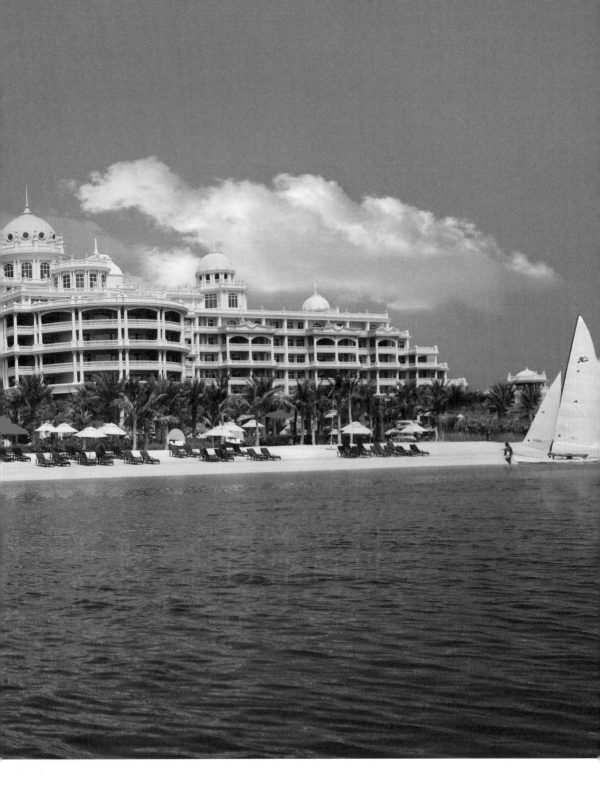

ACKNOWLEDGEMENTS

Writing a book, and especially a book that sums up a whole lifetime of research and discovery, is bound to conjure up vivid memories of the personalities who played their part and got us to where we are today.

My thanks to **Nathalie Bouchon-Poiroux** who accompanied me on my discovery of the world's great traditions of health and beauty. My experience has been all the richer for her enthusiasm, knowledge and confidence. She was at my side at the founding of Cinq Mondes, and still plays a part in its development today.

Sri Sri Ravi Shankar has been much more than a spiritual guide. He brought meaning and lightness to my life, and is ever ready with mischievous but always relevant and lighthearted comments about my spas, as if we saw each other on a daily basis. The depth of his teachings and the kindness and simplicity with which he expresses them are a constant source of inspiration to me.

My friend and supporter, **Galya Ortega**, yoga teacher, therapist and international spa specialist, was an ever-precious asset as the book took shape. Her kindly appreciation was the perfect foil for the demanding artistic sensibilities and perfectionism of our attentive editor **Laure Lamendin**. Thanks too to designer **Benjamin Heuzé** to whom we owe the creative style of the book.

I owe sincere thanks to Doctor **Ghanashyam Marda** who serves as my link between India and Ayurvedic medicine and its application in the Western world. He is among the experts that Cinq Mondes spas constantly call upon, to strengthen team expertise and help formulate our care programs and treatment protocols. It is my wish that all of our treatments should be absolutely authentic and based on the principles of Ayurveda, which is a great tradition and a way of living in its own right. Doctor Ghanashyam Marda is the guarantor of that authenticity.

My research has always linked traditional medicines and herbal remedies with cutting-edge cosmetics science. Along the way, I met **Gérard Redziniak**, doctor in molecular biophysical chemistry, innovator in the field of dermo-cosmetics and the inspiration behind several of our Cinq Mondes products. I greatly appreciate his knowledge and erudition and his generosity in steering Cinq Mondes toward ever-greater achievements in cosmetics innovation.

A big thank-you to **Serge Michenaud**, disciple of Sri Sri Ravi Shankar, who has contributed so much to my understanding of the breathing techniques taught by the master. It was thanks to him that I was able to formalize the founding principles of Sudarshan Kriya – a powerful, energizing and liberating yoga breathing technique.

Special thanks to **Marguerite Laborde** who helped me all along the way as I combed through our Cinq Mondes records in search of treasured images.

Last, but by no means least, thanks to **Arthur** and **Clémentine Poiroux** for having so graciously agreed to let their father immerse himself in many long hours of writing!

Editorial Coordination:
Laure Lamendin

Graphic design and art work:
JusteCiel

Translation from French:
Florence Brutton

Library of Congress Control Number: 2018934208
ISBN: 978-1-4197-3326-0

Printed and bound in 2018 in Portugal
10 9 8 7 6 5 4 3 2 1

ABRAMS
The Art of Books

195 Broadway
New York, NY 10007
abramsbooks.com